Complaints, Litigation and Clinical Errors

This concise book provides readers with practical guidance to help them to both avoid errors and develop robust processes to protect themselves and their patients, as well as dealing appropriately with complaints and litigation, when things do go wrong. Free of complex legal terminology, the book outlines key concepts in medical law and how these may be applied to clinical situations in both hospital and community settings.

Incorporating case law with practical studies, legal information is supplemented by clinical commentaries from a range of specialists representing the perspective of the health care practitioner. The book is essential reading for medical and health students, practising clinicians and allied health care professionals at all levels.

Complaints, Litigation and Clinical Errors

A Practical Guide for Health Care Students and Professionals

Amar Alwitry

Consultant Ophthalmologist
Cataract & Refractive Surgeon
Nottingham, UK

Janine Collier

Executive Partner
Tees Law
Cambridge, UK

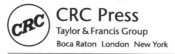

CRC Press
Taylor & Francis Group
Boca Raton London New York

CRC Press is an imprint of the
Taylor & Francis Group, an **informa** business

Designed cover image: Shutterstock image 795328330

First edition published 2024
by CRC Press
2385 NW Executive Center Drive, Suite 320, Boca Raton, FL 33431

and by CRC Press
4 Park Square, Milton Park, Abingdon, Oxon, OX14 4RN

CRC Press is an imprint of Taylor & Francis Group, LLC

ISBN: 978-1-032-01631-3 (hbk)
ISBN: 978-1-032-01627-6 (pbk)
ISBN: 978-1-003-17935-1 (ebk)

DOI: 10.1201/9781003179351

Typeset in Minion
by Deanta Global Publishing Services, Chennai, India

Dedicated to my father who I still miss

Amar Alwitry

Contents

About the authors

Amar Alwitry is a practicing consultant ophthalmologist in the East Midlands and speciality advisor to the Care Quality Commission (CQC). He commenced medicolegal practice after obtaining his master's in medical law and has written three textbooks and two novels. He is father to four children, Max, Toby, Oscar and Safia, and married to Claudia, a GP and aesthetic practitioner. He has an active interest in patient safety and education.

Janine Collier is a partner at Tees Law, a law firm with a recognised top tier medical negligence practice. She studied classics and then law at Cambridge University prior to qualifying as a solicitor in 2001 and has specialised in medical negligence ever since. She is a trustee at Action against Medical Accidents (AvMA), the patient safety charity, and believes in learning from avoidable harm to drive standards in patient safety. She has delivered a number of talks to health care professionals and has had numerous articles published. She is married to Nick and is mother to two children, George and Ben (currently studying medicine!), as well as two dogs, Boo and Winnie!

1

Introduction

We are all well aware that the pressures on the health service in the UK are increasing dramatically. Socioeconomic factors mean that the demand for services is becoming harder to meet and the finances to meet them are becoming stretched. Clinicians are working under unprecedented circumstances and things will go wrong. How they deal with things when they do not go to plan is important. With an abundance of no-win no-fee companies offering services to disgruntled patients the chance of complaints escalating to litigation is higher than ever.

We have a duty of care to our patients to protect them and do everything in our power to preserve their health. They put their trust in us and it is a privilege to serve them. We are human however and things will and do go wrong, resulting in potential harm.

Patients in such circumstances deserve compensation as we have failed them and the law is there to protect them. The law is not just there to catch health care professionals out or to penalise and punish them. The law offers safeguards to us all to protect us and our families, and it should be applied levelly and fairly across all of society.

All those involved in any aspect of delivering health care, from those in nursing or medical careers, students or professional clinicians, those involved in many of the allied medical services, to all administrative staff, have a duty to ensure they are aware of their governance and medicolegal responsibilities. They are also likely to come into the firing line at some stage and be involved in some complaint or even full-blown litigation.

This book seeks to address the why and how of complaints, litigation and clinical errors. It is aimed at all health care professionals regardless of position or experience. It seeks to provide simple, concise and practical advice and information on how to deal with all aspects of the process. It is deliberately not onerous and is not designed as any form of legal text. It should be readable and helpful for the student nurse all the way up to the senior professor in their everyday clinical practice.

The speciality sections address the big specialities, but the principles are the same for all specialities.

DOI: 10.1201/9781003179351-1

The authors hope that this book assists you in understanding how complaints occur and escalate to litigation, provides some information about the litigation process and offers valuable tips and strategies to avoid getting embroiled in what is undoubtedly a very stressful process.

SECTION 1

The law overview

2

The basic principles of the law of medical negligence

The potential causes of action for a claim for medical negligence include:

- *The civil tort of negligence* – this is the most common cause of action.
- *The Law Reform (Miscellaneous Provisions Act) 1943/Fatal Accidents Act 1976* – these Acts apply when the patient has died.
- *The Human Rights Act 1998*[1] – this is most commonly used when psychiatric patients commit suicide but may also be used more generally in cases where there are systemic failures in the system that result in death.
- *Breach of contract* – this is sometimes used when the patient has paid for their health care and may also be used in cases where contractual damages are preferable to compensation in tort.

More rarely used are claims for assault/battery, intentional infliction of harm[2] or death or injury caused as a result of a product defect.[3]

THE TORT OF NEGLIGENCE

Very strict legal tests must be satisfied for any tortious legal claim to be successful.

A failing in the care provided does not automatically constitute grounds for a claim.

Likewise, the fact that a patient suffers an adverse outcome in the course of their health care does not necessarily mean that a claim for negligence will be successful.

The key legal tests are:

1. *There must be a duty of care.*[4]

   A duty of care exists between a patient and a clinician,[5] and that duty arises whenever the clinician provides clinical advice, diagnosis and

DOI: 10.1201/9781003179351-3

treatment.[6] Likewise, a duty exists between those running a health care service and a patient who arrives for treatment, e.g. in an Accident and Emergency Department.[7]

2. *There must be a breach of that duty of care.*

In a clinical context, breach of duty means a failure to act in accordance with the standard of a reasonably competent practitioner[8] in the applicable field of expertise[9] at the time of the incident in question. Lack of experience is not a defence to meeting the standard of a reasonable competent practitioner.[10]

The law recognises that, more often than not, a range of opinion in relation to health care exists. Provided a health care professional is able to demonstrate that they have acted in accordance with a body of opinion that is reasonable, responsible and not plainly wrong and illogical,[11] this is sufficient to constitute a defence.

Examples of breaches of duty often seen in medical negligence claims include:

- Failure to diagnose
- Incorrect diagnosis
- Failure to treat (including delay)
- Incorrect treatment
- Failure to advise appropriately on risks or alternatives
- Poor administration (e.g. failure to follow-up)
- Lack of consent

3. *That breach of the duty of care must cause some harm/injury.*

There must be an adverse outcome (harm/injury) that would not have occurred had it not been for the substandard care.

Different legal tests are available to the court when considering causation, such as:

- *The 'but for' test*: On the balance of probabilities, *but for the breach of duty*, would the injury have occurred?
- *Material contribution*: If there are concurrent causes and it is not possible to prove that the breach of duty was the sole or even main cause of injury, it is sufficient to prove that the breach of duty made a material (more than negligible) contribution to the injury.[12]
- *Material increase to the risk of injury*: In some cases, a material increase to the risk of injury may amount to a material contribution or suffice in its own right to establish causation.

THE PARTIES TO A CLAIM

The person bringing the claim is known as the claimant.

A claim is usually brought by a patient. However, in the case of protected parties, e.g. a child or an adult who lacks capacity, the case can be brought by a 'litigation friend' on their behalf. If the patient has died, the claim can be brought by the personal representative of their estate and/or any dependents.

The person/legal entity against whom the claim is brought is known as the defendant.

If the care is provided by the National Health Service (NHS) in an NHS hospital, then the Trust responsible for that hospital is typically the defendant in any claim. This is because NHS Trusts are vicariously liable for the negligent acts and omissions of their employees.

NHS trusts in England are represented and indemnified by the NHS Resolution, and in Wales, the NHS Wales Shared Services Partnership and Welsh Health Legal Services indemnify and represent the trusts.

If a claim is proven, the NHS bodies should accept full financial liability and not seek to recover any contribution or costs from the health care professional involved.

If a claim arises from treatment provided in a private hospital, the claim is usually brought against an individual clinician. Claims arising out of nursing care, however, are more likely to be brought against the hospital.

All clinicians should have indemnity insurance, and when a claim is intimated, the relevant medical defence organisations (MDOs) ought to provide cover. However, indemnity issues can arise, and health care professionals working in private settings are advised to carefully check the terms of any indemnity insurance policy to ensure that cover will be provided in the event of a claim (and any exclusions that may apply) and that the limit of indemnity on the policy will be sufficient to pay not only any compensation that may be awarded to a patient but also their legal costs. If a claim falls outside the indemnity insurance policy, the MDO withdraws indemnity and/or the indemnity is insufficient, health care professionals will find themselves personally liable to satisfy any court judgement that may be obtained.

If the care is provided by a general practitioner (GP), the GP is often the defendant in the proceedings. If multiple GPs are involved in the care and/or the care is provided by others employed by or working for the practice, the practice may be the defendant. This is because the practice is vicariously liable for its employees[13] and has non-delegable duties,[14] and the partners are liable for other partners.[15]

Historically, claims against GPs were indemnified by MDOs, such as the Medical Defence Union or the Medical Protection Society. However, the NHS now provides indemnity for primary care in relation to treatment provided on or after 1 April 2019, and as such, claims arising from incidents after 31 March 2019 are represented and indemnified by the NHS Resolution, and this liability no longer falls to MDOs.

The same NHS indemnity applies to other health service practitioners working under contracts for services, e.g. dental practitioners, pharmacists and optometrists.

COMPENSATION

In law, the sole remedy that can be court-ordered in a civil claim for medical negligence is financial compensation. Remedies such as punitive, criminal or disciplinary actions are not available through the civil court system.

The principle of the law is that compensation should, as closely as possible, put the patient in the same position they would have been in had the negligence not occurred.[16]

Awards of compensation take into account:

- Physical pain; psychological suffering, such as anxiety, fear and embarrassment; and reduction in enjoyment of life resulting from the injury.

- Any past expenses and losses that have been incurred as a result of the injury. Most commonly, this includes loss of earnings, care and attendance, aids and equipment, travel expenses, medical treatment, therapies, prescription charges and sundry expenses.

- Future losses and expenses, if any, arising from the injury, such as loss of future earnings capacity, future case management and care, additional accommodation costs, transport and travel expenses, medical treatment and therapy costs, and miscellaneous and sundry expenses.

In some cases, there may also be awards for loss of satisfaction and enjoyment in carrying out a particular job ('loss of congenial employment'), disadvantage on the labour market and costs associated with professional deputyship, among others.

The claimant must provide evidence to prove the compensation claimed.

OTHER REMEDIES

Although compensation is the only legal remedy available to a claimant in a civil claim, it is the primary motivator for a claimant to bring the claim in just 6% of cases. More commonly, the primary reasons are to prevent similar incidents from happening to others (35%), to hold clinicians to account (21%), to obtain a detailed investigation and explanation of the incident (10%), to receive an apology (10%) and frustration with the handling of the incident (9%).[17]

Therefore, it is not uncommon for a claimant to seek an apology and/or assurances that there will be improvements in patient safety resulting from changes in policies and procedures when seeking to resolve a claim, particularly if a mediation takes place.

NOTES

1. Rabone v Pennine Care NHS Foundation Trust [2012] UKSC 2.
2. Wilkinson v Downton [1897] 2 QB 58; Rhodes v OPO [2015] UKSC 32.
3. Consumer Protection Act 1987.
4. There must be *proximity* between the claimant and the defendant and the *foreseeability* of harm, and it must be fair, just and reasonable for a duty of care to be imposed. Caparo Industries plc v Dickman [1990] 2 AC 605.
5. Robinson v Chief Constable of West Yorkshire Police [2018] UKSC 4.
6. R v Bateman (1925) 94 LJKB 791.
7. Carney v Croydon Health Services NHS Trust [2018] UKSC 50.
8. The legal 'test is the standard of care of the ordinary skilled man exercising and professing to have that special skill. A man need not possess the highest expert skill: it is well established law that it is sufficient if he exercises the ordinary skill of an ordinary competent man exercising that particular art'. Bolam v Friern Hospital Management Committee [1957] 1 WLR 582.
9. Meiklejohn v (1) St George's Healthcare NHS Trust (2) Homerton University Hospital NHS Foundation Trust [2014] EWCA Civ 120.
10. FB v Princess Alexandra Hospital NHS Trust [2017] EWCA Civ 334.
11. Bolitho v City & Hackney Health Authority [1998] AC 232.
12. Bailey v Ministry of Defence [2008] EWCA Civ 883; Williams v Bermuda Hospitals Board [2016] UKPC 4.
13. Cox v Ministry of Justice [2016] UKSC 10; Mohamud v Wm Morrison Supermarkets plc [2016] UKSC 11; Barclays Bank PLC v Various Claimants [2020] UKSC 13; Wm Morrison Supermarkets plc v Various Claimants [2020] UKSC 12; Hughes v Rattan [2022] EWCA Civ 107 Cox.
14. Woodland v Essex County Council [2013] UKSC 66; Nyang v G4S Care & Justice Services Ltd [2013] EQHC 3946 (QB); GB v Home Office [2015] EQHC 819 (QB).
15. s9, Partnership Act 1890. See also Dubai Aluminum Co Ltd v Salaam [2003] 2 AC 366.
16. Lim Poh Choo v Camden and Islington Area Health Authority [1980] AC 174; Wells v Wells [1999] 1 AC 345; Whittington Hospital NJHS Trust v XX [2020] UKSC 14; Swift v Carpenter [2020] EWCA Civ 1295.
17. Behavioural Insights into Patient Motivation to Make a Claim for Medical Negligence, NHS Resolution, August 2018.

3

Consent

A basic principle of law is that a patient must give their consent to medical treatment.

When it is alleged that there has been a failure to properly advise on risks or reasonable alternative treatments, the cause of action is likely to be negligence. If it is contended that there has been a failure to obtain consent at all, the cause of action is assault/battery.

To give valid consent, a patient must have capacity, and consent must be informed and given voluntarily.

DOES THE PATIENT HAVE CAPACITY TO GIVE CONSENT?

The Mental Capacity Act 2005 (MCA) sets out a statutory test for mental capacity to be applied in England and Wales. In the context of medical care, to be able to make a decision, the patient must be able to:

- Understand the information relevant to the decision
- Retain that information
- Use or weigh it as part of a decision and
- Communicate their decision effectively by any means

The MCA makes clear that patients should be presumed to have capacity unless it can be established otherwise.

Capacity is both time- and decision-specific.

INFORMED CONSENT

In 1985, the House of Lords determined that the health care professional decides what information to provide when warning patients of the risks inherent in the treatment being proposed.[1] However, over the following years, the case law moved away from paternalistic medicine towards patient autonomy and doctors working in partnership with patients to make decisions about their health care.[2] A raft

DOI: 10.1201/9781003179351-4

of professional guidance has addressed the nature and extent of the information that a patient should be given to ensure that they are giving informed consent.

In 2008, the General Medical Council (GMC) issued the guidance 'Consent: Patients and Doctors Making Decisions Together',[3] and in 2013, the GMC guidance 'Good Medical Practice'[4] instructed doctors to:

- Work in partnership with patients
- Listen and respond to their concerns and preferences
- Give patients the information they want or need in a way they can understand
- Respect patients' rights to reach decisions with doctors about their treatment and care

MONTGOMERY

In 2015, the Supreme Court reconsidered the duty of care a doctor owes a patient when advising on medical treatment in the landmark case *Montgomery v Lanarkshire Health Board*.[5] Known as the 'Montgomery standard', it is the legal benchmark for informed consent in the United Kingdom (UK).

The case involved a pregnant woman, Nadine Montgomery. Ms Montgomery was of slight build and had diabetes. Diabetes increases the risk of a large baby and the risk of shoulder dystocia during a vaginal delivery by 9–10%. Ms Montgomery was concerned about the risks associated with a vaginal delivery and raised these with her obstetrician, McLellan. It was Dr McLellan's policy

> not routinely to advise diabetic women about shoulder dystocia as, in her view, the risk of a grave problem for the baby was very small, but if advised of the risks of shoulder dystocia women would opt for a caesarean section, which was not in the maternal interest.[6]

Thus, Ms Montgomery delivered vaginally. The baby was large, and he suffered from shoulder dystocia and oxygen deprivation during delivery, as well as consequent serious disabilities.

It was alleged that Dr McLellan failed to properly inform Ms Montgomery of the risks of giving birth to a large baby, given that she was a small woman with diabetes, and that there was a failure to advise on the alternative to vaginal delivery, such as a caesarean section, which could have prevented the baby's injuries.

Ruling in favour of Montgomery, the UK Supreme Court stated that **doctors have a duty to take reasonable care to ensure that patients are aware of any material risks involved in any recommended treatment and of any reasonable alternative or variant treatments**. Such information must be given in terms the patient can understand.

The Montgomery case is significant because it shifted the focus of informed consent from a paternalistic doctor-centred model, where the doctor is the primary decision-maker who makes decisions on behalf of the patient, to a more patient-centred approach, where the patient has the right to be fully informed of the material risks associated with their care and to make their own decisions about their treatment (or refusing treatment). Patients should be actively involved in the decision-making process and empowered to make decisions based on their individual circumstances and preferences.

A 'therapeutic exception' provides that a doctor may withhold information if they reasonably consider that its disclosure will cause the patient psychological harm to a degree that outweighs the benefits of informing them. However, the Supreme Court made it very clear that this is not to be abused.

Nevertheless, the possibility of this exception presents significant legal difficulties for health care professionals. Litigation is a likely consequence of the use of the therapeutic exception, and health care professionals should ensure that, if they use it at all, their reasons should be documented at the time. If contentious issues are involved, legal advice should be sought.

WHAT IS A MATERIAL RISK?

The test of materiality is based on what a reasonable person in the patient's position would consider significant. Under this test, a risk is considered material if, at the time in question:

- The risk should reasonably have been known to the health care professional[7]

- The risk is one that a reasonable person in the patient's position would consider significant or if the doctor is or should reasonably be aware that the particular patient would attach significance to it[8] and

- The doctor knows or ought reasonably to know that the patient would be likely to attach significance to the risk

Materiality is fact- and case-sensitive. For example, an ophthalmic procedure carrying a negligible risk of sight loss in one eye is likely to be material to a patient who has already lost sight in the other eye. It may be less material to a fully sighted patient.

GENERAL MEDICAL COUNCIL GUIDANCE

In 2020, the GMC issued the updated guidance 'Decision Making and Consent'. The guidance outlines seven core principles:

- All patients have the right to be involved in decisions about their treatment and care and be supported to make informed decisions if they are able.

- Decision making is an ongoing process focused on meaningful dialogue: the exchange of relevant information specific to the individual patient.

- All patients have the right to be listened to and to be given the information they need to make a decision and the time and support they need to understand it.

- Doctors must try to find out what matters to patients so they can share relevant information about the benefits and harms of proposed options and reasonable alternatives, including the option to take no action.

- Doctors must start from the presumption that all adult patients have capacity to make decisions about their treatment and care. A patient can only be judged to lack capacity to make a specific decision at a specific time and only after assessment in line with legal requirements.

- The choice of treatment or care for patients who lack capacity must be of overall benefit to them, and decisions should be made in consultation with those who are close to them or advocating for them.

- Patients whose right to consent is affected by law should be supported to be involved in the decision-making process and to exercise choice if possible.

This guidance is intended to support doctors in their conversations with patients. Following it will help doctors ensure that patients give informed consent to their care. It provides advice on:

- What to tell a patient when talking about risks

- What to do if the patient refuses to hear information that is relevant

- What to do if the patient may lack the capacity to make a decision

- What to document

WHO SHOULD CONSENT THE PATIENT?

In the UK, typically, the health care professional who is responsible for the patient's care should lead the discussions. This may mean doctors, nurses, dentists or other health care professionals.

The 2020 GMC guidance allows for the delegation of part of the decision-making process, but the guidance makes it clear that the doctor should carefully consider whether it is appropriate to delegate. If the responsibility is delegated, that person should be suitably trained and competent; should have sufficient knowledge of the proposed treatment plan and its benefits and risks, as well as alternative options; must have the skills to discuss consent with the patient; and should feel competent to ensure that the patient gives informed consent. If part of the decision-making process has been delegated, the doctor is still responsible for ensuring that the patient has been given the information they need to make the decision, has had time and support to consider it and has given their consent before treatment or care is provided.

WHEN IS THE RIGHT TIME TO CONSENT A PATIENT?

Consent is a continuum. It begins at the first consultation.

If the decision is for an elective procedure, the patient should give consent that is documented well in advance of any procedure. Furthermore, the patient should be given a 'cooling-off' period to deliberate, consider their treatment options and do their homework.

In the UK, there is no specific time limit for the validity of patient consent to treatment. Patient consent is an ongoing process and can be withdrawn at any time, even after treatment has started.

In certain cases, such as for treatments that carry significant risks, where a patient's capacity to consent is in question or where circumstances have changed in a way that significantly alters the patient's condition, material risks or any other aspect of treatment, renewed consent should be sought and appropriately documented in the medical records.

GETTING INTO THE RIGHT MINDSET

Consent is a patient's to give, not a doctor's to take. There is no routine consent. *A signature on a consent form does not equate to consent.*

Facilitating a patient to give valid consent takes time.

Health care professionals should get to know their patients and find out what matters to them, personally and professionally, so that they can understand their patients' needs, values and priorities that influence their decision making, as well as their concerns and preferences about the options and their expectations about what treatment or care may achieve.

All information given should be tailored to the patient, and discussions should take place in terms the patient can understand. Visual or other aids may be helpful, for example, to put a patient-specific risk in the context of general population risk.

The language used should be objective, clear and unbiased, and the health care professional should be truthful, open and honest during the discussion. The health care professional should ensure that the patient understands the information provided and has the opportunity to ask questions.

WHAT INFORMATION SHOULD BE GIVEN TO THE PATIENT?

The health care professional should explain several key pieces of information to the patient to help them give informed consent, including:

- *Diagnosis*: The diagnosis and the condition being treated
- *Treatment options*: The various treatment options available, including their risks and benefits
- *Prognosis*: The likely outcome of the condition without treatment
- *Risks and benefits*: The risks and benefits of the proposed treatment, including the likelihood and severity of potential side effects
- *Alternative treatments*:
  (a) Any alternative treatments available that are within the knowledge of a reasonably competent clinician at the time and are an accepted practice and an appropriate treatment, not just a 'possible' treatment[9]
  (b) Their risks and benefits
- *Recovery time*: How long it will take the patient to recover from the treatment
- *Cost*: Any costs associated with the treatment
- *Consent*: The consent process and ensuring that the patient understands that they have the right to refuse treatment

More detail is provided in paragraphs 10 and 13 of the GMC guidance 'Decision Making and Consent'.

DOCUMENTING CONSENT

Documenting the consent process in the patient's medical records is important to ensure that there is a clear record of the discussions conducted and decisions made. This helps ensure that the patient's wishes are respected and that health care professionals have a clear understanding of the patient's medical history and treatment preferences.

Health care professionals should record:

- The capacity assessment, if the patient's capacity to consent was assessed
- The decision-making process, including the discussions conducted with the patient, the information provided, any questions asked and any concerns or preferences expressed by the patient
- The patient's decision, including the date and time of the decision
- The risks and benefits of the proposed procedure that were discussed, including any potential complications and their likelihood and severity
- Any alternative treatments discussed, including their risks and benefits
- Concerns or objections, if the patient expressed any
- The identity of the person who provided the information

It is good practice not only to document these in a written clinical note but also in correspondence to the patient's GP, and the patient should receive a copy.

In the case of *Malik*,[10] the clinician concerned did not keep handwritten notes or typed notes of the consent consultation. HHJ Blair QC commented:

I was taken aback by his practice of simply dictating a letter to his patient's GP after an outpatient clinic appointment to relay the details of his patient's current symptoms, recording his clinical assessment, giving his opinion as to appropriate treatment(s) but omitting to state what advice has been given about the risks and benefits of the avenue(s) open to the patient. This is a practice which it seems to me is fraught with risks of being unable confidently to answer important questions many years later without having the benefit of a contemporaneous set of detailed notes.

CONSENT IN SPECIAL CIRCUMSTANCES

In certain circumstances, it may be difficult for a health care professional to obtain consent to be able to treat the patient. For example:

- *Children*: Children under the age of 16 are generally not considered legally competent to make their own decisions about medical treatment. In these circumstances, consent must be obtained from a parent or legal guardian. However, if the child is deemed to be competent to make their own decision, their consent can be obtained instead.[11]

- *Adults lacking capacity*: If the patient lacks the capacity to make decisions about their medical treatment, the health care professional must seek consent from someone who has the legal authority to make decisions on their behalf. This may be a family member, an appointed representative or the Court of Protection.

- *Emergencies*: In emergency situations where the patient is unable to provide consent, treatment may be given without consent if it is in the patient's best interests.

- *Mental health conditions*: If the patient has a mental health condition that affects their decision-making capacity, the health care professional must determine whether the patient has the capacity to give consent to treatment. If the patient lacks capacity, consent must be sought from someone who has the legal authority to make decisions on their behalf.

In all special circumstances, the health care professional should ensure that they obtain valid consent or authority to treat the patient. This may involve following specific legal and ethical guidelines and consulting with other health care professionals and legal experts when necessary.

NOTES

1. Sidaway v Board of Governors of the Bethlem Royal Hospital [1985] AC 871.
2. Rogers v Whitaker [1992] HCA 58; 175 CLR 479; Pearce v United Bristol Healthcare NHS Trust [1999] ECC 167; Chester v Afshar [2004] UK HL 41.
3. https://www.gmc-uk.org/-/media/documents/GMC-guidance-for-doctors---Consent---English-2008---2020_pdf-48903482.
4. https://www.gmc-uk.org/-/media/documents/good-medical-practice-english-20200128_pdf 51527435.pdf.
5. Montgomery v Lanarkshire Health Board [2015] UKSC 11.
6. https://www.supremecourt.uk/cases/docs/uksc-2013-0136-press-summary.pdf.
7. Duce v Worcestershire Acute Hospitals NHS Trust [2018] EWCA Civ 1307 (7 June 2018).
8. A v East Kent Hospitals University NHS Foundation Trust [2015] EWHC 1038 (QB) (31 March 2015); Tasmin v Barts Health NHS Trust [2015] EWHC 3135 (QB) (30 October 2015); Spencer v Hillingdon Hospital NHS Trust [2015] EWHC 1058 (QB).
9. Bayley v George Elliot Hospital [2017] EWHC 3398.
10. Malik v St George's University Hospital NHS Foundation Trust [2021] EWHC 1913 (QB).
11. Gillick v West Norfolk and Wisbech AHA 1986 provided that children under the age of 16 can consent to their own treatment if they fully appreciate what is involved.

4

Criminally negligent manslaughter

Criminally negligent manslaughter (or gross negligence manslaughter, as it is mostly referred to in English law) is a form of involuntary manslaughter. This crime is different from murder, where there is intent to kill or cause grievous bodily harm.

In the context of health care, it is exceptionally rare for a health care professional's behaviour to be deemed criminal. The crime of gross negligence (medical) manslaughter arises when death occurs as the result of truly, exceptionally bad health care.

THE LEGAL TESTS

Gross negligence manslaughter is when a death occurs as a result of a grossly negligent but otherwise lawful act or omission by a health care professional.

In 1994, an anaesthetist called Adomako was convicted of gross negligence manslaughter. Dr Adomako did not notice that a patient's oxygen pipe had become disconnected during an operation. Consequently, the patient died. The judge stated the test for gross negligence manslaughter,[1] which includes the following:

- There must be a duty of care.

  A health care professional always owes a duty of care to their patients.

- The health care professional must have breached that duty of care.

  Per the (civil) law of negligence, in a clinical context, breach of duty means a failure to act in accordance with the standard of a reasonably competent practitioner,[2] in the applicable field of expertise,[3] at the time of the incident in question.

DOI: 10.1201/9781003179351-5

- That breach must have caused the death of the patient.

  This element of the offence requires that the breach of duty caused the death of the patient, but it does not have to be the sole or even principal cause. It merely must have more than minimally caused the death.

  In cases of omission potentially leading to death, as opposed to an act, the prosecution must prove that the negligent failure to act was a substantial cause of death.

- A serious and obvious risk of death was foreseeable.

  The jury must find that a reasonable person in the health care professional's position at the time would have foreseen a serious and obvious risk of death, not merely a risk of injury or even serious injury.

  While a health care professional's subjective awareness may be relevant when assessing the obviousness of the risk of death, this test remains objective in nature.

- The breach of duty was so serious in all the circumstances that it should be judged criminal.

  The prosecution must prove that the circumstances were such that a reasonable person in the health care professional's position would have foreseen a serious and obvious risk of death arising from their act or omission and that the breach of duty was reprehensible and so far below the expected standard of someone in their position (with the same qualifications, experience and responsibilities) that it amounted to a crime.

The definition of gross negligence in R v Adomako is as much maligned as it is seemingly circular because it seeks to define criminal conduct by asking the jury to determine whether the conduct is criminal without defining what constitutes criminal conduct. Thus, it can be hard for a health care professional to know whether their conduct will be deemed criminal or not.

The judge did provide some examples of what might constitute a criminally serious breach, such as:

- Indifference to an obvious risk of injury to health

- Knowledge of the risk of injury to health at the outset but a determination to run the risk nevertheless

- Knowledge of the risk of injury to health and an intention to avoid it but coupled with such a high degree of negligence in attempting to avoid that injury that a jury deems it a charge of criminally serious breach, as necessary

The best advice to a health care professional is to do their job at the highest standard to avoid the criminality of their conduct ever being called into question. However, the law recognises that all professionals are human and may make mistakes: 'Mistakes, even very serious mistakes, and errors of judgment, even very serious errors of judgment, are nowhere near enough for a crime as serious as manslaughter to be committed'.[4]

HOW IS AN INVESTIGATION TRIGGERED?

Usually, a criminal investigation is triggered by the coroner referring the case to the police for investigation, although families can also ask the police to look into the circumstances of death. The Crown Prosecution Service (CPS) considers whether it is in the public interest to prosecute the relevant medical professional and whether prosecution is a proportionate response.

WHO DECIDES THE CASE?

A jury decides the case in a criminal court.

To secure a conviction, the jury must be satisfied beyond all reasonable doubt that the individual or trust committed the crime of gross negligence manslaughter.

PENALTIES

The offence of gross negligence manslaughter carries a maximum sentence of life imprisonment.

EXAMPLES OF GROSS NEGLIGENCE MANSLAUGHTER CONVICTIONS

Some examples of gross negligence manslaughter convictions include:

- In 2007, Stevenson, a GP, injected Marjorie Wright with six times the correct dose of diamorphine for a migraine. He admitted to manslaughter but was spared jail. His 15-month jail term was suspended for 2 years.
- An 80-year-old patient, Winifred Bowman, died at the Royal Sussex County Hospital due to complications from a hip operation in 2005. Nurse Amaro was found guilty of gross negligence manslaughter in 2008 after it was discovered that she failed to properly monitor Bowman's vital signs. She was sentenced to 30 months in prison.
- In 2010, Ubani, a German doctor working for an out-of-hours service in Cambridgeshire, administered a lethal dose of diamorphine to a patient named David Gray. Dr Ubani was found guilty of gross negligence manslaughter and was sentenced to 9 months in prison.

- Hadiza Bawa-Garba, a trainee doctor, was found guilty of gross negligence manslaughter in 2015 when she failed to diagnose and treat sepsis, resulting in the death of a 6-year-old boy, Jack Adcock. She was sentenced to 2 years in prison, which was later reduced to a suspended sentence on appeal.
- In 2017, Richard Neale, a pharmacist, was found guilty of gross negligence manslaughter in the death of a young girl who was given ten times the pre-scribed dose of an epilepsy drug. Mr Neale was responsible for dispensing the medication and failed to notice the error before it was administered. He was given a 9-month suspended prison sentence.

CORPORATE MANSLAUGHTER

Corporate manslaughter was established in UK law via the Corporate Manslaughter and Corporate Homicide Act 2007, which, for the first time, allowed for companies and organisations to be found guilty of corporate man-slaughter as a result of serious management failure resulting in a gross breach of a duty of care.

As a result, gross negligence manslaughter cases can no longer be brought against companies and organisations.

The threshold for establishing corporate liability for manslaughter is very high. It must be proven beyond all reasonable doubt that:

- The defendant is a qualifying organisation.
- The defendant owed a duty of care to the deceased.
- The defendant grossly breached that duty of care.
- Senior management played a substantial role in that breach.
- The breach caused or contributed to death.

In the medical context, NHS trusts may face criminal prosecution for corporate manslaughter if a patient dies as a result of gross negligence. If found guilty, the health care trust may be fined and/or ordered to take steps to remedy any defi-ciencies in its health and safety policies, systems or practices.

EXAMPLES OF CORPORATE MANSLAUGHTER CONVICTIONS

Few health care trusts in the UK have faced prosecution for corporate man-slaughter. However, examples include:

- Maidstone and Tunbridge Wells NHS Trust was prosecuted in 2009 follow-ing an outbreak of *Clostridium difficile* that caused the deaths of 5 patients and contributed to the deaths of 22 others. The trust pleaded guilty to charges of corporate manslaughter and was fined £750,000.

- In 2013, the Mid Staffordshire NHS Foundation Trust was found guilty of corporate manslaughter in relation to the deaths of patients who received poor care at Stafford Hospital between 2005 and 2009. The trust was fined £200,000.
- In 2021, Southern Health NHS Foundation Trust was prosecuted in relation to the death of a patient, Conor Sparrowhawk, who drowned in a bath in its care. The trust pleaded guilty to charges of corporate manslaughter, was fined £2 million and received an additional fine of £950,000 for breaching health and safety laws.

Prosecutions of health care trusts for corporate manslaughter are rare, and most cases involving health care providers tend to result in charges of gross negligence manslaughter rather than corporate manslaughter.

NOTES

1. R v Adomako [1995] 1 A.C. 171.
2. The legal 'test is the standard of care of the ordinary skilled man exercising and professing to have that special skill. A man need not possess the highest expert skill: it is well established law that it is sufficient if he exercises the ordinary skill of an ordinary competent man exercising that particular art'. Bolam v Friern Hospital Management Committee [1957] 1 WLR 582.
3. Meiklejohn v (1) St George's Healthcare NHS Trust (2) Homerton University Hospital NHS Foundation Trust [2014] EWCA Civ 120.
4. R v Misra [2004] EWCA Crim 2375.

5

Bawa-Garba and the use of reflections in court

The case of R v Bawa-Garba [2016] EWCA Crim 1841 led to widespread debate about the working conditions and pressures faced by health care professionals in the UK. It has also shaped the use of a health care professional's reflections in legal proceedings and has sparked a debate about whether a doctor's reflections should be considered confidential and whether they may be used against them in court.

On 4 November 2015, before judge and jury, Hadiza Bawa-Garba, a trainee doctor, was convicted of the gross negligence manslaughter of Jack Adcock and was sentenced to 2 years imprisonment, which was later reduced to a suspended sentence on appeal. The nurse on duty at the time, Isabel Amaro, was also convicted of the same offence, but the ward sister, Theresa Taylor, was acquitted.

In Dr Bawa-Garba's fitness to practise hearing in 2017, the Medical Practitioners Tribunal Service (MPTS) found her guilty of multiple charges of professional misconduct, including failing to properly assess and monitor Jack. The MPTS concluded that Dr Bawa-Garba's actions fell significantly below the standards expected of a competent and conscientious junior doctor and that her failings contributed to Jack's death. The GMC applied for Dr Bawa-Garba to be struck off the register, but the MPTS rejected this, saying that erasure would be disproportionate given the mitigating and aggravating factors. Instead, they imposed a 12-month suspension on her ability to practise. The GMC appealed the decision, arguing that suspension was insufficient to maintain public confidence in the medical profession. In 2018, the appeal succeeded, and Dr Bawa-Garba's suspension was replaced with the decision to strike her name from the medical register. Following a crowdfunding campaign, Dr Bawa-Garba appealed the decision to erase her name from the register. The appeal was successful and the decision overturned, with Dr Bawa-Garba being reinstated in the medical register with a one-year suspension.

DOI: 10.1201/9781003179351-6

WHAT ARE REFLECTIONS?

Doctor's reflections are a key component of the appraisal and revalidation process in the UK. Reflection is the process of thinking about and analysing one's own experiences and actions, with the aim of identifying areas for improvement and learning.

In the medical profession, doctors are encouraged to reflect on their clinical practice, including their interactions with patients, colleagues and other health care professionals. This can involve thinking about how they approached a particular case, what they learned from the experience and how they might do things differently in the future.

Reflection can take many forms, including written reflections, recorded audio or video, discussions with colleagues or mentors and participation in peer reviews or quality improvement activities. Doctors are required to document their reflections as part of their appraisal and revalidation process, and these reflections are used to inform their ongoing professional development.

Reflection is seen as an important tool for improving patient care and preventing errors in the medical profession. By encouraging doctors to think critically about their practice and learn from their experiences, reflection can help promote a culture of continuous improvement and innovation in health care.

THE USE OF DR BAWA-GARBA'S REFLECTIONS IN COURT

Contrary to several reports, Dr Bawa-Garba's e-portfolio reflections statement on the case were *not* presented to the court or the jury during her trial for gross negligence manslaughter.[1]

However, Dr Bawa-Garba's duty consultant, O'Riordan, did include *his* thoughts following his meeting with Dr Bawa-Garba to discuss the incident and learnings in his witness evidence. Attached to his evidence was a trainee encounter form not signed by Dr Bawa-Garba. The trainee encounter form was not a component of Dr Bawa-Garba's e-portfolio and did not contain any admission of guilt or liability. Moreover, it was not referred to by either the CPS or the defence during the trial and, therefore, was not considered by the jury.

In fact, the court was clear from the start that reflections were irrelevant to the facts of the case and that no weight should be given to any remarks documented after the event.

THE USE OF DR BAWA-GARBA'S REFLECTIONS IN THE FITNESS TO PRACTISE HEARING

In Dr Bawa-Garba's case, some personal reflections – though not the e-portfolio statement – were shared with the panel to show her remediation efforts.

In her reflections, Dr Bawa-Garba acknowledged a number of mistakes that were made during Jack's care, including misinterpreting test results and not escalating his care to a more senior doctor in a timely manner.

THE GENERAL MEDICAL COUNCIL'S POSITION

The case provoked widespread debate about the confidentiality of a doctor's reflections and the possibility of their use against them in court.

This led to a review of the General Medical Council's (GMC) guidance on reflective practice, with the aim of clarifying the use of reflections in legal proceedings. The GMC stated that doctors' reflections should be considered private and confidential and should not be used as evidence in legal proceedings. The MPTS also stated that doctors should be able to reflect openly and honestly on their cases without fear of legal consequences in order to promote a culture of learning and improvement in the medical profession.

THE CURRENT POSITION

The GMC has confirmed that it does not request reflective notes from doctors to investigate concerns in relation to them. However, an individual may choose to offer them as evidence of their insight into their practice.

In a civil legal case, all written materials, including reflections, are potentially disclosable in the context of litigation, and there is no legal privilege shielding reflections or e portfolios from disclosure.

ADVICE TO DOCTORS

Reflective practice is a crucial aspect of professional development, as it allows for ongoing learning, practice improvement and the cultivation of self-awareness.

Doctors are recommended to work with their supervisors to determine the best approach to reflecting on their experiences and documenting this process.

Documenting reflections in a way that is meaningful and relevant could include writing in a diary, completing reflective forms or templates and discussing experiences with supervisors.

When documenting reflections:

- Keep it confidential: Reflective practice is a personal and confidential process, and doctors should ensure that their reflections are not shared without their permission.
- Patient details in any reflections and feedback should be entered anonymously so that individuals cannot be identified from what is written.
- Be honest: Reflections should be honest and include both positive and negative experiences to promote learning and growth.
- Focus on learning: Reflections should focus on learning and improvement (learning outcomes) rather than blame or criticism, while factual details should be recorded elsewhere.
- Use a structured approach: Some doctors find it helpful to use a structured approach to document reflections, such as the Gibbs reflective cycle and the Johns reflective framework.

If uncertain about the admissibility of their reflections in a legal context, doctors should seek legal advice.

For further details, doctors should consider 'The Reflective Practice Guidance'[2] for doctors and medical students.

NOTES

1. https://www.gmc-uk.org/-/media/documents/20180419-factsheet---dr
-bawa-garba-case-final_pdf-74385491.pdf.
2. https://www.gmc-uk.org/-/media/documents/dc11703-pol-w-the-reflec-
tive-practioner-guidance-20210112_pdf-78479611.pdf.

SECTION 2

Regulatory bodies

6

The General Medical Council

The GMC is a regulatory body in the UK that is responsible for setting and maintaining the standards of medical education, training and practice.

WHAT IS THE ROLE OF THE GENERAL MEDICAL COUNCIL?

The GMC plays a crucial role in maintaining public trust in the medical profession and ensuring that doctors in the UK are qualified, competent and practicing to a high standard to ensure that patients receive safe and effective care from their doctors.

The GMC has several responsibilities, including:

- *Setting standards*: The GMC sets standards to ensure that medical students and doctors in the UK receive the necessary education and training to provide safe and effective care to patients. This includes the standards for medical schools, the requirements to practice as a doctor and the training and assessment needed to maintain registration with the GMC.
- *Registration and licensing*: The GMC maintains a register of all licensed doctors in the UK. To practice medicine in the UK, a doctor must be registered with the GMC. The GMC also issues licences to doctors who meet its standards and requirements.
- *Fitness to practise*: The GMC investigates complaints and concerns about doctors' behaviour or performance. This includes cases of professional misconduct, poor performance and health issues that may affect a doctor's ability to practice safely. If necessary, it can take disciplinary action against doctors who breach its standards. This may include suspending or revoking a doctor's registration if necessary.
- *Promoting good medical practice*: The GMC promotes good medical practice by providing guidance and advice to medical students, doctors, patients and the public. It also publishes ethical guidance for doctors on issues such as confidentiality, consent, end-of-life care, best practice in clinical care and communication with patients.

DOI: 10.1201/9781003179351-8

WHAT ARE THE OBLIGATIONS OF DOCTORS TO THEIR PATIENTS?

The GMC defines the duties and obligations of doctors to their patients in its guidance document 'Good Medical Practice' (GMP).[1] The GMP guidelines emphasise the importance of doctors placing their patients' needs at the centre of their practice and maintaining high standards of professionalism and ethical conduct.

Some key obligations include:

- *Putting patients first*: Doctors must prioritise their patients' care. This means providing good quality care, treating patients with respect and dignity and acting in their best interests.
- *Communicating effectively*: Doctors must listen to their patients and communicate effectively with them.
- *Obtaining informed consent*: Doctors should explain diagnosis and treatment options clearly to patients and ensure that they have the information they need to be able to make informed decisions about their care. They should respect patient autonomy.
- *Working collaboratively*: Doctors must work collaboratively with patients and other health care professionals to provide the best care. This includes respecting the roles and expertise of others and working in partnership with patients to develop care plans that meet their needs.
- *Maintaining trust*: Doctors must be honest and trustworthy in all their professional dealings and act with integrity.
- *Continuing professional development*: Doctors must keep their knowledge and skills up to date and ensure that they are providing care based on the latest evidence and best practice.
- *Maintaining professional boundaries*: Doctors must maintain appropriate professional boundaries with their patients, avoiding any behaviour that may be interpreted as exploitative or abusive.
- *Raising concerns*: Doctors should raise concerns if they believe that patient safety or care is being compromised.

The document 'Good Medical Practice' provides more detailed guidance on these and other issues.

WHAT IS THE DIFFERENCE BETWEEN BREACH OF DUTY AND BREACH OF THE GENERAL MEDICAL COUNCIL'S GOOD MEDICAL PRACTICE GUIDANCE?

Breach of duty for the purposes of a legal claim for medical negligence and breach of GMP are two distinct, albeit related, concepts.

Breach of duty refers to a situation in which a health care professional fails to provide an appropriate standard of care to a patient. A legal concept, it is typically assessed based on the objective standard of what a reasonably competent health care professional would have done in similar circumstances. A breach of duty may occur when a doctor fails to diagnose or treat a patient appropriately or when they make a mistake during a procedure.

Breach of GMP, by contrast, refers to a situation in which a doctor violates the ethical and professional standards defined by the GMC in their GMP guide. This may include failing to maintain appropriate professional boundaries with patients, failing to communicate effectively with patients or colleagues and engaging in behaviour that is considered unprofessional or unethical.

While breach of duty and breach of GMP may overlap in some situations, a breach of GMP does not necessarily equate to a breach of duty and vice versa. For example, a doctor who breaches GMP by failing to communicate effectively with colleagues may not have breached their duty of care if they still provided appropriate medical treatment. Similarly, a doctor who breaches their duty of care by providing substandard treatment may not have breached their duty of care if they were acting in good faith and following ethical principles.

A breach of duty may lead to legal action in a civil court, with the claim being brought by the patient or their family.

A breach of GMP may result in regulatory action by the GMC.

GENERAL MEDICAL COUNCIL INVESTIGATIONS

The GMC's role is to protect patients by ensuring that doctors meet the GMP standards. The focus is on whether a doctor is fit to practise as a doctor.

Some examples of issues that the GMC may investigate include:

- Complaints from patients or their families about the care provided by a doctor, including allegations of negligence or unethical behaviour
- Concerns raised by colleagues or employers about a doctor's conduct, performance or health
- Criminal convictions or charges against a doctor
- Breaches of the GMC's professional standards or ethical guidelines
- Failure to meet the requirements for continuing professional development or revalidation

Fitness to practise investigations are not intended to punish doctors for past mistakes or behaviour but rather to ensure that there are no concerns that would undermine public confidence in the profession or put patients at risk should a doctor continue to practise. Therefore, it is rare for the GMC to consider isolated mistakes in patient care, particularly when the individual has complied with all professional and ethical values and behaviours expected of a doctor when an adverse incident has occurred, has explained what has happened and the likely effects, has done what they could to put matters right, has apologised and has demonstrated that they have learned from the incident and taken steps to minimise the risk of the error being repeated.

Any concerns about a doctor's fitness to practise should be raised as soon as possible. Apart from exceptional circumstances, the GMC will only consider complaints raised within 5 years of the incident.

The GMC aims to complete investigations as quickly as possible, and it has set targets for the time to complete various stages of the investigation process. For example, the initial assessment of a complaint should be completed within 5 working days, while an investigation must be concluded within 12 months. The length of an investigation can vary depending on the complexity and seriousness of the case, the amount of evidence to be gathered and assessed and the availability of witnesses and experts.

While an investigation is ongoing, to protect the public and maintain public confidence in the medical profession, the GMC may refer the case to the MPTS for an interim orders tribunal hearing and seek interim orders, such as a suspension or conditions on a doctor's registration. An example of such a restriction is to stop the doctor from operating unsupervised or without seeking agreement on the necessity of the surgery with a colleague. Interim orders are regularly reviewed, and the GMC must apply to a court to extend them beyond certain time limits.

Depending on the severity of the case and the findings of the investigation, a number of potential outcomes may follow a GMC investigation, such as:

- *No further action*

    If the GMC finds no evidence of serious misconduct or incompetence, it may decide to take no further action and close the case.

- *Advice or guidance*

    The GMC may provide advice or guidance to the doctor, such as recommending changes to their practice or providing education and training.

- *Warning*

    If there are no concerns that the doctor poses a risk to the public, but the GMC considers that their behaviour or performance was below the standard expected, the GMC may issue a formal warning to the doctor, which will be recorded on their registration and may be taken into account in any future investigations or proceedings. Warnings are published on the GMC website for 2 years and can be disclosed to employers on request.

    If the doctor refuses to accept a warning, the GMC will refer the matter to an Investigation Committee hearing, which can impose the warning or decide to take no further action.

- *Undertakings*

    In more serious cases, but ones that fall short of requiring the doctor to be struck off the register, the GMC may require the doctor to provide undertakings to the GMC, such as agreeing to certain conditions on their practice or behaviour. Undertakings allow doctors to address concerns about their practice while avoiding the need for formal disciplinary action and ensure that patients are protected while the doctor takes steps to improve their practice.

Undertakings may include restrictions on the type of work that the doctor can do, where they can work, how their work will be supervised and any additional training that should be undertaken. The doctor will usually be required to keep the GMC informed of any changes to their practice. The GMC will liaise with the doctor's employer and responsible officer to make sure the doctor honours this agreement.

Undertakings are published on the GMC's website and will remain visible for 10 years after the expiry of the undertaking.

Undertakings are legally binding, and failure to comply with the terms can result in further action by the GMC, including a referral to the MPTS for a formal hearing.

- *Referral to the MPTS for a hearing*

THE MEDICAL PRACTITIONERS TRIBUNAL SERVICE

The MPTS is an independent adjudication body that is responsible for holding hearings and making decisions on cases referred to it by the GMC. It is responsible for ensuring that the fitness to practise of doctors is assessed fairly and impartially.

The MPTS operates independently from the GMC and comprises independent medical and lay members. The panel is chaired by a legally qualified person who is not a doctor.

The tribunal has the power to make a range of decisions, including imposing sanctions on a doctor's registration or ordering them to take steps to improve their practice. Its courses of action include:

- *Dismissing the case*

If the MPTS finds that there is no case to answer or that the allegations are unfounded, it can dismiss the case and clear the doctor of any wrongdoing.

- *Ordering the doctor to undertake training or retraining*

The MPTS can require the doctor to undertake additional training or retraining to improve their knowledge, skills or practice.

- *Issuing warnings*

The tribunal may issue a warning to the doctor if they have breached professional standards or if there are concerns about their fitness to practise.

- *Imposing sanctions on the doctor's registration*

  This can include suspending the doctor's registration, placing conditions on their registration or removing them from the register ('erasure').

  The doctor's registration may be suspended for a specified period, which means they cannot practise as a doctor during that time.

  The tribunal may impose conditions on the doctor's registration, such as requiring them to work under supervision or limiting the types of patients they can treat.

  In the most serious cases, the doctor's name may be erased from the medical register, which means they can no longer practise as a doctor in the UK.

- *Referring the case for a criminal investigation*

  If the tribunal believes that the allegations against a doctor are serious enough to warrant a criminal investigation, it can refer the case to the appropriate authorities.

Any decisions can be appealed through the courts.

NOTE

1. https://www.gmc-uk.org/-/media/documents/good-medical-practice---english-20200128_pdf-51527435.pdf.

7

The Parliamentary and Health Service Ombudsman

The Parliamentary and Health Service Ombudsman (PHSO) is an independent body in the UK that investigates complaints about government departments, public services and the NHS in England.

WHAT IS THE ROLE OF THE OMBUDSMAN?

Its key role is to hold public services to account by providing an independent and impartial service for complaints that have not been resolved through other channels.

The key responsibilities and functions of the PHSO include:

- *Investigating complaints*: The PHSO has the power to investigate complaints about a wide range of issues, including maladministration, service failure and inadequate professional conduct.
- *Making recommendations*: After completing an investigation, the PHSO makes recommendations to the organisation or service provider involved, as well as to government departments and other stakeholders. These recommendations are designed to improve services, prevent similar problems from happening in the future and provide redress for those affected by poor service.
- *Raising awareness*: The PHSO raises awareness of the importance of good public service by publishing reports and highlighting issues and trends that emerge from its investigations. It also works with other organisations to promote good practice and improve service delivery across the public sector.
- *Providing guidance and advice*: The PHSO provides guidance and advice to members of the public who are considering making a complaint, as well as to organisations and service providers on how to improve their complaint handling processes.

DOI: 10.1201/9781003179351-9   35

WHAT ARE THE OBLIGATIONS OF PROFESSIONALS TO THE OMBUDSMAN?

Health care professionals in the UK have certain obligations to the PHSO in relation to complaints made about them or the services they provide. These obligations include:

- *Cooperating with investigations*: Health care professionals have a duty to cooperate fully with any investigations carried out by the PHSO. This includes providing information and documentation as requested, attending interviews or hearings and answering questions truthfully.
- *Providing accurate and complete information*: Health care professionals must provide accurate and complete information when responding to complaints or inquiries from the PHSO. This includes providing information about their own actions and decisions and the policies and procedures of the health care organisation they work for.
- *Taking complaints seriously*: Health care professionals have a duty to take complaints made against them or their organisation seriously and to respond to them in a timely and appropriate manner. This includes conducting internal investigations, providing explanations or apologies and taking steps to address any issues that are identified.
- *Implementing recommendations*: When the PHSO makes recommendations as a result of an investigation, health care professionals have an obligation to implement these recommendations to the best of their ability. This may involve changes to policies, procedures or practice and may require additional training or resources.
- *Maintaining professional standards*: Health care professionals have a duty to maintain professional standards at all times and to act in the best interests of their patients. This includes providing high-quality care, communicating effectively with patients and their families and treating everyone with dignity and respect.

Overall, the PHSO ensures that complaints are handled in a fair and transparent manner and that the public can have confidence in the health care system. By complying with the obligations listed, health care professionals can help the PHSO fulfil its important role in promoting accountability and improving public services.

COMPLAINT INVESTIGATIONS

The PHSO is not the first point of contact for complaints and will only consider investigating health care complaints after all other avenues have been exhausted and if certain criteria are met. These criteria include:

- The complaint must be made by or on behalf of someone who has received treatment or care from the NHS or other public health bodies in England.
- The complaint must have already gone through the relevant NHS complaints procedure. Before the PHSO can investigate a complaint, the complainant must have gone through the health care provider's complaints process and received a final response. If the complainant is not satisfied with the response or a response is not received within 6 months, they can escalate to the PHSO.
- The complaint should be about a matter of injustice or hardship resulting from improper conduct by staff or maladministration or service failure by an NHS organisation.
- The complainant must have suffered, or be likely to suffer, as a result of the maladministration or service failure.
- The complaint must be about an issue that has not already been investigated by the PHSO, unless new evidence has emerged.
- The complaint must be about an issue that is within the PHSO's jurisdiction.
- The complaint must not be subject to legal proceedings, unless the PHSO has agreed to investigate alongside the legal process.

If these criteria are met, the PHSO will consider the complaint and decide whether to investigate.

The PHSO does not investigate all cases and will prioritise investigations into complaints that are serious in nature, such as those involving serious harm or death, those where wider public interest issues are raised and those where it believes it can make the biggest difference.

The PHSO may decline to investigate if the complaint is considered to be frivolous or vexatious or if there is insufficient evidence to suggest that maladministration or service failure has occurred.

Typically, the PHSO will only consider complaints made within one year from the date of the final response from the health care provider, although some discretion is retained in relation to time limits.

The PHSO logs all complaints it receives about NHS-funded services so that if it receives a similar complaint about the organisation or sees a pattern from a number of complaints, it may be able to raise this with the organisation in the future.

If the PHSO does investigate, it looks at each case individually.

The process includes an initial assessment in which the PHSO assesses the complaint and issues raised to ensure that they are within its remit and that all other avenues for complaints have been exhausted. If otherwise, the PHSO may advise the complainant to pursue other options.

The PHSO then investigates the complaint by reviewing all the information gathered and considering whether there has been any maladministration, service failure or improper conduct by staff in the health care provider. The investigation may also include seeking expert opinions and advice.

Once the investigation is complete, the PHSO prepares a draft report of its findings and conclusions. The health care provider and the complainant are given an opportunity to respond to the report before it is finalised.

Then the PHSO issues a final report containing the findings of the investigation, any recommendations for actions and any remedies or compensation that the PHSO considers appropriate. Remedies include requiring the health care organisation to apologise to the complainant, calling for changes to prevent such an incident from happening again and reviewing procedures. While the PHSO can recommend compensation for inconvenience, distress and expenses incurred, this is not designed to replace the legal process for claiming compensation if there is negligence. When suggesting financial payments, to help them identify how much ought to be paid, the PHSO refers to its 'severity of injustice scale' and payments previously recommended as part of its casework.

Thereafter, the PHSO monitors the health care provider's response to the report and ensures that the recommendations are implemented. The PHSO may also follow-up with the complainant to ensure that they are satisfied with the outcome.

The length of time it takes for the PHSO to investigate a complaint can vary depending on the complexity of the case and its workload. Some complaints may be resolved quickly, while others may take several months or even years to investigate fully.

8

The Care Quality Commission

The Care Quality Commission (CQC) is the independent regulator of health and social care services in England. It has the power to take enforcement action against providers who do not meet the required standards of care.

WHAT IS THE ROLE OF THE CARE QUALITY COMMISSION?

Its main role is to ensure that health and social care services provide safe, effective, compassionate and high-quality care to those who use them.

The CQC sets standards and inspects health and social care providers, such as hospitals, GP surgeries, care homes and domiciliary care agencies. It monitors, inspects and regulates services to ensure that they meet the standards and takes action if they do not.

The CQC also provides information and guidance to the public about health and social care services. Ultimately, the CQC aims to improve the quality of care for all people who use health and social care services in England.

WHAT ARE THE OBLIGATIONS OF PROFESSIONALS TO THE CARE QUALITY COMMISSION?

Professionals who work in health and social care services have certain obligations to the CQC. These obligations are designed to ensure that the CQC can monitor and regulate services effectively and that providers are held accountable for the care they provide. Some of the key obligations include:

- *Registration*: Professionals who provide health and social care services must register with the CQC. These include individual practitioners, such as doctors and nurses, and organisations, such as hospitals and care homes.
- *Compliance with standards*: Professionals have an obligation to ensure that the services they provide meet the CQC's standards for quality and safety.

DOI: 10.1201/9781003179351-10

This includes ensuring that the care they provide is effective, responsive, caring and well led.

- *Cooperation with inspections*: Professionals are required to cooperate with CQC inspections and provide access to information and records as requested from the start. They are also expected to be open and transparent with the CQC about any issues or concerns that arise.
- *Reporting incidents*: Professionals have a duty to report certain incidents to the CQC, such as serious injuries or deaths that occur as a result of the care provided.
- *Continuous improvement training*: Professionals are expected to engage in continuous improvement activities to ensure that they are providing the highest quality of care possible. These include training and development, quality improvement initiatives and other activities aimed at improving the care they provide.

CARE QUALITY COMMISSION INVESTIGATIONS

The CQC may undertake investigations into concerns and complaints about health and social care services in England.

Investigations can be initiated in a number of ways, including through complaints from service users, their families or representatives; staff members; whistle-blowers and other regulatory bodies. The investigations aim to assess the quality of care provided by the service and to identify any areas where improvements need to be made.

The investigation process can vary, but typically, the CQC conducts an initial assessment to determine the level of risk to the safety or well-being of the service users and to decide whether to take any immediate action. This assessment may involve gathering additional information or speaking to the people involved.

Based on the findings from the initial assessment, the CQC may decide to launch a full investigation. If an investigation is launched, the CQC informs the service provider of the investigation and the concerns raised. It plans the investigation by identifying the scope and objectives, deciding on the methods and tools to be used and determining the timeline. Usually, there is an on-site investigation, which includes interviews with service users, staff, management and other relevant parties; reviewing documents and records; and observing the care being delivered.

The CQC then analyses their findings and evaluates the service against the relevant regulatory standards. It prepares a draft report that summarises the investigation's findings, identifies areas of good practice and areas where improvements are needed, and makes recommendations. The draft report is shared with the service provider, and they are then given an opportunity to provide feedback and comments. After taking these into account, the CQC publishes its final report, which is available to the service provider, the service's commissioners and the public. This report includes any areas where the service has failed to meet the required standards and any actions that need to be taken to improve the quality of care provided.

If the service is found to be failing to meet the required standards, the CQC may take enforcement action, which includes:

- *Warning notices*: The CQC may issue a warning notice to the service provider outlining the areas of concern and the requirements to address them.
- *Improvement notices*: If the service fails to make the required improvements, the CQC may issue an improvement notice, which legally requires the service to take specific actions within a set time frame.
- *Prosecution*: In cases when there are serious or persistent breaches of the regulations, the CQC may decide to take legal action against the service provider or its individuals, which can lead to a fine, payment of a victim surcharge and costs or imprisonment. All fines are paid to the Treasury.
- *Cancellation of registration*: In extreme cases, the CQC may cancel the service provider's registration, preventing them from operating the service.

The service provider is required to address any areas of concern identified by the CQC. It may also be required to provide regular updates to the CQC on the progress made towards making improvements.

As of February 2023, the CQC has brought 86 prosecutions against various service providers and individuals. Only three sentences have been imposed and only against individuals. One received a suspended sentence and was ordered to perform community service and attend an offenders' course. Another was disqualified from acting as a company director for 5 years, while the third was given a 6-month community order and required to do 80 hours of unpaid work.[1]

The largest fine imposed was £2,533,332. This arose from the prosecution of the Dudley Group NHS Foundation Trust. The Trust pleaded guilty to a Regulation 12 charge of failing to provide safe and effective care. Two patients died from sepsis in separate incidents, and the CQC had repeatedly raised with the trust its failure to adequately monitor for sepsis prior to these deaths.

CARE QUALITY COMMISSION INSPECTIONS

CQC inspections are different from CQC investigations. A CQC inspection is a routine evaluation process to assess the quality of care provided by the health or social care services provider, to determine whether the service is meeting the required standards of quality and safety and to identify any areas where improvements can be made.

Inspections are usually planned in advance and carried out by a team of CQC inspectors. The process varies depending on the type of service being provided.

Before the inspection, the CQC sends a notification to the service provider informing it of the date and time of the inspection. The provider is also asked to provide information about the service, including its policies, procedures and patient records.

The inspection team visits the service provider's premises to observe the care provided to patients or other service users. It also reviews the service's policies and procedures, interviews staff members and talks to patients and their families to gather feedback about the service.

Feedback is given to the service provider during and after the inspection. During the inspection, the inspection team may provide feedback on any areas where improvements can be made. Afterwards, the team provides a summary of its findings, including a rating for the service. Ratings range from 'outstanding' to 'inadequate'.

The CQC produces an inspection report based on the findings. The report includes a summary of the service's strengths and areas for improvement, as well as its rating. Such reports are published on the CQC's website and are used to inform the public about the quality of care provided by the service and to help patients and their families make informed decisions about their care. An organisation's reputation and survival may be significantly affected by unfavourable inspections by the CQC. This may result in the provider losing funding, commissioning, public trust, patients and customers or even facing closure.

NOTE

1. https://www.cqc.org.uk/about-us/how-we-do-our-job/prosecutions.

9

The coroner

Coroners are specialist judges who investigate and provide explanations for certain deaths. They are also required to carry out an investigation if they have been notified of a possible discovery of treasure (Treasure Act 1996).

As an independent judicial office, coroners operate separately from the government to ensure impartiality in verdicts rendered and freedom from political interference.

The role was established in 1194. In England and Wales, local authorities appoint a legally qualified solicitor or barrister as a senior coroner, who may be assisted by area coroners and assistant coroners. Coroners are supported by coroner's officers employed by the police or local authorities.

There are currently 83 jurisdictions of coroners in England and Wales, and they are locally funded.

THE ROLE OF A CORONER

The coroner investigates and determines the causes and circumstances of certain types of deaths, which include:

- Violent or unnatural deaths
- Suspicious deaths
- Deaths where the cause is unknown
- Deaths in state detention, e.g. in custody
- In very rare circumstances, where there is an exceptionally high-profile case or aa fundamental legal reason

WHO REFERS DEATHS TO THE CORONER?

Not all deaths are referred to the coroner. In cases where the death was expected and the cause of death is clear, such as natural death due to a known medical condition, a referral to the coroner may not be required.

DOI: 10.1201/9781003179351-11

In general, medical practitioners, usually doctors, are the ones who report such deaths as those listed above to the coroner, and indeed, they are required to do so.

In addition to medical practitioners, the police, a funeral director or a concerned family member can also report a death to the coroner. The coroner may also become involved in cases where a person has gone missing and their whereabouts and welfare are unknown.

WHAT HAPPENS ONCE A DEATH IS REFERRED TO THE CORONER?

The coroner will consider all deaths referred and:

- If the cause of death is clear to the coroner, then a medical certificate is signed and sent by a doctor to the registrar, who registers the death. The coroner provides the registrar with a certificate of confirmation that a post-mortem is not required.
- If the cause of death is not clear, then the coroner requests a post-mortem, which no other party can object to. Once the post-mortem is completed and if no further investigations are required to determine the cause of death, the coroner releases the body and notifies the registrar of the cause of death.
- If the cause of death is not clear after the post-mortem or if the individual died a violent/unnatural death or in police custody/prison, then the coroner opens an inquest (a public inquiry into the death). Interested persons can request that an inquest be held, but the coroner decides whether the case fits the criteria for one.

WHAT IS AN INQUEST?

An inquest is the coroner's investigation into a death. The coroner seeks to answer four questions during an inquest investigation:

- Who was the deceased?
- Where did the deceased die?
- When did the deceased die?
- How did the deceased die?

The purpose of an inquest is not to apportion blame; it is a fact-finding investigation.

The coroner must follow the inquest rules as stated in the Coroners and Justice Act 2009 and the Coroners (Inquests) Rules 2013. However, each inquest is different, and the practices of the coroners vary across different local authorities.

In R (Parkinson) v HM Senior Coroner for Kent, the court clarified that if there is reason to believe that a death may have resulted from medical staff failing to meet their professional obligations, an Article 2 inquest must be held to comply with Article 2 of the European Convention on Human Rights (right to life).

Juries are only required in an inquest in exceptional cases; for example, if the death occurred while the deceased was detained under the Mental Health Act 1983.

HEALTH CARE PROFESSIONALS AND THE CORONER'S COURT

The coroner typically grants certain parties interested person (IP) status for an inquest.[1] IPs can include immediate family members, hospital trusts and care homes. Having IP status gives the individual/organisation the right to participate in the inquest and receive disclosure if requested. IPs can question witnesses and make submissions to the coroner on issues that they believe should be investigated; thus, it is common for IPs to seek legal representation at the inquest. The running order for questioning a witness is the coroner, the family of the deceased and then other IPs.

As well as deciding which witnesses are called to provide evidence for an inquest (live or read), the coroner may also request, and subsequently disclose to IPs if relevant, further evidence. The evidence obtained can include medical records and hospital trust investigation reports.

Health and social care service professionals who were involved in providing the deceased's treatment may be called as witnesses during the inquest. They may be requested by the coroner to prepare written statements and attend the inquest as live witnesses to provide evidence. Alternatively, they may only be requested to provide written evidence to be read at the inquest.

Whether writing a statement for an Inquest or providing live evidence, it is essential for the health care professional to keep in mind the key obligations that all witnesses have to the coroner's court, including:

- Their overriding duty is to the court.
- The evidence provided must be knowledge obtained in a professional capacity, as far as possible, and based on notes and clinical records made at the time in question. It should be made clear whether the written statement was based on clinical records or recollection.
- Any written evidence submitted by a health care witness should be that witness's recollection of events.
- The coroner will, if necessary, instruct expert witnesses to advise the court; therefore, the health care professional should provide factual evidence, unless their opinion is specifically requested.
- If providing live evidence, the health care professional should prepare beforehand by rereading their written statement.
- Evidence is provided under oath and must be factual, accurate, clear and honest. It should be unbiased and objective. Criminal sanctions may be

imposed for not being honest, withholding information and providing misleading evidence.

- Questions must be answered truthfully and accurately. If an answer to a
  question is unknown, then the witness should say so.
- If an opinion is asked of the witness, it should only be provided if it is within
  the witness's expertise to do so. If it is not within the witness's expertise, then
  this should be stated.
- Health care professionals are required to follow their professional regulatory
  rules.

Health care providers called to provide live evidence at inquests may be asked
questions regarding the scope of the inquest, such as:

- Information about the deceased's medical history
- The deceased's treatment plan and the reasons for it
- Any medications the deceased was taking
- Any relevant test or investigation results
- Any procedures or surgeries the deceased underwent
- Why the concerns were not escalated according to hospital protocols
- The reasons for discharging the patient

Evidence from health care professionals is often essential for the coroner, or jury
if present, to be able to answer the four questions and conclude the inquest.

WHAT HAPPENS AT THE END OF THE INQUEST?

At the end of the inquest, the coroner provides their conclusion, which is then
written on the record of inquest and the individual's final death certificate. If a
jury has been called, then they provide the details for the record of inquest.

Conclusions in health care inquests may take various forms, depending on the
facts of the case, and may include one of the following:

- *Natural causes*: The cause of death was due to natural causes, such as a medical condition or disease.
- *Accident or misadventure*: The death was the result of an accident or unin-
  tended consequence, which may or may not have involved some degree of
  fault or error.
- *Neglect*: The death was due to a lack of care; for example, the health care
  provider failed to provide the necessary level of care to the patient, resulting
  in harm or death.
- *Unlawful killing*: The deceased was unlawfully killed, either intentionally or
  through gross negligence.
- *Lawful killing*: The death was caused by the deliberate actions of another
  person or persons, but the actions were deemed necessary and lawful.
- *Suicide*: The deceased took their own life and intended to do so.

- *Narrative*: This is a detailed description of the events leading up to the death, highlighting any issues that contributed to the death.
- *Short-form*: This is a brief statement that summarises the key findings of the inquest.
- *Open*: There is insufficient evidence to determine the cause of death.

The conclusion is not a finding of guilt or liability but a determination of the cause and circumstances of the death.

When reaching their conclusion, the coroner takes into account all available evidence, including medical records, relevant guidelines, protocols and regulations, and witness statements, as well as any other relevant information, such as contributory factors that may have played a role; for instance, underlying health conditions or external factors. Conclusions are drawn on the balance of probabilities, and the coroner applies legal tests that have been established by case law and legislation.

WHAT HAPPENS AFTER THE INQUEST?

Following an inquest, in cases where the coroner is concerned about the risk of further deaths in similar circumstances to the individual(s) in question, the coroner makes a prevention of future deaths report (also known as a Regulation 28 Report) to the appropriate person or authority, such as the health and safety executive of a hospital trust. The recipient has 56 days to reply in writing, with details of actions that have been taken or will be taken or an explanation as to why no action will be taken, to prevent similar deaths in the future.

NOTE

1. Section 47 of the Coroners and Justice Act 2009.

SECTION 3

Special circumstances

10

The junior doctor

Being a junior doctor can be daunting, tiring, draining, rewarding and challenging. The learning curve is steep, and stress is an ever-present companion. Doctors
often move from one speciality to another and, when they first enter a new post,
they have no experience at all in managing the specialist patients they see. They
are literally thrown in at the deep end and expected to swim with very little aid.
Lack of experience, however, does not mean lack of responsibility, and often, they
are at the coalface of dealing with patients and in the line of fire of clinical errors.
The same issues apply for students in all our health care fields and settings.

RESPONSIBILITIES OF A JUNIOR DOCTOR

Currently, the training of a junior doctor starts with a 2-year foundation period
after completing their primary medical degree. The foundation period is designed
to help the doctor adjust to the responsibilities and workload in a safe and secure
environment, supported by senior doctors and their team to prevent error and
harm. Sadly, the senior doctors and team are often at full stretch and the safety
net can have significant holes. The junior doctor must avoid falling into these
holes, and if they do fall, they need to be able to clamber back up again.

The pressure is intense, and maintaining the standard of care can be difficult
at times, particularly when backup is not provided. Needless to say, many mistakes are made in these 2 years. Not only can these mistakes lead to harm, but
they can also have a significant detrimental effect on the doctor's self-esteem,
confidence and career progression.

Historically the junior doctor used to pride themselves on not calling their
senior for advice; however, this means courting the risk of harm. You will not be
thanked for not asking and the consequences of harm to the whole team.

The most common errors the junior doctor may make are:

- **Failure to obtain consent**: Each department has different procedures and
  paperwork. While the themes of the consent forms are usually similar,
  details can vary due to the nature of the surgery/procedure/treatment. For
  instance, some procedures require verbal consent, while others require

written consent. In some departments, such as paediatrics and psychiatry, the law requires specific standards of the consent giver, and the doctor should be aware of these. It is imperative that all junior doctors familiarise themselves with the consent details before participating in the consent process.

A junior doctor should never obtain consent for a procedure they are not well versed in. The Royal College of Surgeons states:

> Ensure that consent is obtained either by the person who is providing the treatment or by someone who is actively involved in the provision of treatment. The person obtaining consent should have clear knowledge of the procedure and the potential risks and complications.

Consent is not only documentation but also an interactive process with two-way communication. One size does not fit all, and patients are each unique in their needs, circumstances and attitudes to risk. Ideally, health care professionals obtaining consent should have specific training and it is reasonable to delegate consent responsibilities as long as the appropriate training is given and protocols followed.

The more junior the clinician the more robust the process must be. It is all too easy to fall foul of an allegation that 'the junior doctor just got me to sign the consent form but did not really understand what I was having done and couldn't answer my questions'.

- **Lack of knowledge of important legal issues**: Theoretically, junior doctors are taught about medicolegal issues and legal terms before qualification; however, that education is often inadequate. According to a survey performed in 2008 on junior doctors from three UK hospitals, most junior doctors' knowledge of legal and ethical principles in health care lacks depth.[1] For example, among the 100 doctors surveyed, almost all knew what an enduring power of attorney entailed, but their knowledge of the Assisted Dying Bill was not sufficient. In fact, the doctors admitted a lack of understanding of legal issues.

Junior doctors may face litigation for simply not knowing the correct legal framework. The law regarding critical patient care, end-of-life care and chronic pain patient care can be tricky. The treatment of each type of patient is not the same and is often guided by protocols based on unique conditions. For obvious reasons, not following these protocols means any treatment will be considered wrong, no matter the good intention. These rules apply to all doctors and health care professionals who undertake invasive procedures.

Remember that in the vast majority of situations the procedure will be carried out without issue; however, when things do not go to plan then they inevitably wish to attribute blame and assert that they would never have proceeded with treatment if they had been properly informed of the risks. The junior is an easy target, and so it is vital that everything is done 'by the book'.

- **Providing the wrong treatment to a patient**: Any doctor or health care professional can make mistakes, regardless of how long they have been flaw-lessly practising. Being inexperienced inevitably increases the risk of making a clinical error. While a senior doctor or consultant is usually in charge of the treatment plan, the junior doctor is often the one who implements it after the ward round has moved on. Perceived minor procedures may be delegated to doctors who are not completely confident about them but feel pressured into impressing the boss. Mistakes such as performing the wrong procedure or the correct procedure at the wrong site, using the wrong instruments or simply forgetting a step are all potential grounds for litigation and will not ingratiate the trainee with the senior team. If uncertain about a procedure, no matter how minor it is, the junior doctor should always ask for help from a senior doctor; that is what they are there for. Reflection and awareness of one's limitations are a vital part of practice.

- **Medication errors**: Medication errors constitute a major cause of litigation against doctors. The most common errors that junior doctors make regard-ing medication usually relate to two types of mistakes: knowledge-based and rule-based.[2] Knowledge-based mistakes are prescribing an incorrect drug or dosage, prescribing drugs that are antagonistic or whose interaction produce serious adverse effects, prescribing the wrong timing of the dosage, not pre-scribing antibiotics for the proper duration, etc. Rule-based mistakes are not checking drug allergies before prescribing drugs like penicillin, not checking whether the patient had already been given similar drugs, etc. These gener-ally occur due to a lack of experience or having just enough experience that they fall into an 'automatic thinking' pattern when prescribing medication. Lack of time and rushing through jobs are also common themes. This is in tune with Ryan et al., who found that 'the majority of self-reported errors (250, 49.2%) resulted from unintentional actions. Interruptions and pressure from other staff were commonly cited causes of errors'.[3]

Obviously it is desirable to avoid both types of mistakes. The first step is to immediately note any instruction or drug given by the senior. If the junior doc-tor does not know the spelling or mishears the patient's name/instruction, they should always ask. When caring for a new patient, their medical records should be read carefully before prescribing any new medications or changing existing ones. Inadvertent cessation of a current medication can be just as detrimen-tal as commencing an inappropriate new drug. If there is any doubt about a patient's medical history or allergies, the junior doctor must check again with their consultants, senior staff or the pharmacist before prescribing any medication to them. If in doubt, the patient or even their GP should be asked for information that is lacking.

Each prescription should have the name of the drug, dose, frequency, before/after meal instruction and finishing date written in a clear, legible script. In case of a verbal prescription (e.g. in an emergency situation, such as shock or asphyxia), the name and dosage of the drug should be clearly stated and written down at the earliest convenience, with the date and time of the entry recorded.

- **Error in patient or drug identification**: This is another common mistake among junior doctors, who are new to high-volume and high-pressure departments with quick patient turnover; for example, emergency or general medicine. Adopting a few habits, such as checking both the patient's name and identification card when prescribing any medication and matching a patient's description with their drug chart before writing on it, will help avoid these mistakes entirely. There may be multiple patients with the same name or patients from the same family under a doctor's care. Medications should always be checked, including the content, dosage, generic name, route of transmission and expiration date, before they are administered to patients. This is something that should be ingrained and undertaken by medical students all the way until the day before retirement.

- **Failure to diagnose or assess a patient properly**: A very common factor in allegations of negligence are assertions that the junior doctor failed to take an accurate history or appropriately and correctly diagnose a patient. Although the junior doctor is rarely responsible for the definitive diagnosis, they are usually asked to make a provisional diagnosis until a senior review occurs. This may be the next morning and therefore can be the source of harm if incorrect. Furthermore, juniors are often responsible for presenting patient histories and examination findings to their seniors, which are the bases of diagnoses. This communication issue can lead to incorrect diagnoses or even conflict among the health care team as to what and what was not discussed/relayed.

- **Documentation**: The importance of documentation cannot be stressed enough. All steps must be documented, including any changes made to the dose/frequency and treatment. All treatment changes should be carried out after they are documented in the clinical record to avoid confusion and provide a timeline of care.

As the record will most likely face detailed scrutiny in case of a complaint or litigation, all notes must be legible, comprehensive and contemporaneous. The urge to omit any minor detail may later present itself as missing information or failure to assess/determine that discredits the doctor and undermines credibility. Record keeping is a vital element of the junior doctor's role. Juniors in any team are an easy target for blame and so they should protect themselves by diligent and detailed documentation.

- **Miscommunication**: Communication is a multifaceted process that includes both verbal and nonverbal cues, along with written and electronic mediums. Lack of prompt reply, prompt relay or initiative to question any confusing orders results in harm and potential litigation.

Doctors must also consider the doctor–patient communication gaps and how they can affect the patient. Sometimes, a little effort might be needed to communicate with patients who are from different cultural backgrounds, have language barriers and have different personalities and educational levels. The latest recommendation is to follow the situation, background, assessment, recommendation (SBAR) technique for uneventful handovers.[4]

Doctor–doctor miscommunication is a more common scenario than most would like to admit. Instructions are easily misheard due to masks, accents, an emergency department rush or a crowded room. Overdose and mistreatment litigation have been noticeably increasing lately due to mistaking similar-sounding words, such as 15 mg/kg and 50 mg/kg, when both parties were wearing masks.[5] Failure of proper information relay during patient handover is another common and easily preventable cause. According to in-depth surveys, simply notifying the oncoming doctor of which patients to see first, who needs to be referred or test reports that need immediate evaluation (head injury CT, X-ray for RTA, blood work for shortness of breath cases, etc.) is enough to avoid most communication gaps.[6] Note that all actions are taken by the junior doctor, and the information they access must be noted in detail to avoid proven guilt in court.

Patients can fall through the gap and be left untreated/unattended because they have not been passed on to an incoming clinician. Such harm is indefensible and will lead to conflict as to who is to blame, the doctor/nurse leaving the shift or the incoming one. It is a joint responsibility and in both parties' interests to ensure a robust process is followed.

Lack of teamwork between junior doctors and nurses causes equal harm, if not more. A study of 33 clinical mishap cases attributed 63.6% to poor collaboration, 42.4% to poor leadership and 48.5% to lack of coordination.[7] In short, miscommunication between medical personnel can have a devastating effect on a patient's health.

- **Breaking doctor–patient confidentiality**: The confidentiality between a doctor and their patient is enshrined, even after death. Sharing any information regarding a patient can result in disciplinary action and even litigation, depending on how sensitive or harmful the information may be and whether any harm occurred. Any discussion outside work must either be generalised or about a hypothetical case. Conversations in lifts and hospital restaurants or at the nurse's station can be overheard and lead to significant complaints.

Note that any competent child is entitled to the same rights as an adult. Also, the name of a patient is considered confidential, as well as the details.

There are certain circumstances where patient confidentiality can be breached; for example, if there is evidence of suspected illegal activity or an infectious or transmissible disease (e.g. COVID-19 and measles). Junior doctors should not consider breaking confidentiality; such decisions should be referred to seniors.

The UK government requires all doctors and medical professionals to adhere to the UK General Data Protection Regulation (GDPR).[8] The GDPR requires a standard data protection policy to be set up to prevent patient data theft or loss. This protection includes both digital and paper records. For example, all digital records should be password protected, and all paperwork must be kept in locked cupboards.

WHO TAKES THE BLAME?

During their work, the junior doctor mostly follows a senior's orders and cares for patients as a proxy for the named consultant responsible for the patient. While some mistakes are their own (e.g. patient identification, procedural error and failure to check the medication), they are rarely in charge of making definitive decisions regarding serious management choices.

Junior doctors are generally not involved in private patient care; therefore, they are not usually sued as individuals.

When complaints occur, the person at the coalface faces scrutiny, and that is often the junior doctor. In a utopian health care setting, the senior doctor magnanimously assumes the blame for their team. As captain of the ship, they should do so to some degree; however, self-preservation inevitably comes into play.

Whether the junior or senior doctor is to blame, the hospital, trust or GP practice defends any claim or complaint; thus, the wider organisation/NHS shoulders the financial burden. It is human nature to try to avoid blame, and attempts to avoid this blame will vary depending on the individual.

A key question is where the blame lies on an individual basis. From a logical point of view, it should be the consultant in charge, as they are responsible for their team. Any failing among their team may be due to poor training, poor supervision or poor organisational factors, and the consultant should take responsibility for these issues. Sadly, this is not the case, and often, the blame focuses on the most available scapegoat, i.e. the junior doctor.

If there is no contemporaneous documentation of instructions or discussions, then it is the senior's words against the junior's. If the senior claims they instructed the junior doctor correctly, there is very little the junior can say in their defence. The senior doctor might assert that they were not told a vital piece of information and that had they been told, they would have managed the patient differently.

An example of the issues a junior can face is starkly highlighted by the Hadiza Bawa-Garba case. Dr Hadiza Bawa-Garba was a registrar in a UK hospital's children's assessment unit (CAU). On the day the patient, Jack Adcock, was admitted, she was the sole doctor running the entire CAU due to rota gaps and the on-call consultant being absent. The patient presented with dehydration and vomiting and was soon found to have metabolic acidosis. Dr Bawa-Garba correctly prescribed tests and fluid replacement; however, according to the consultant, she did not 'stress' to him the need to review the patient. There was also an IT failure in the hospital, which led to delayed test results. Nevertheless, Dr Bawa-Garba correctly prescribed antibiotics after the chest X-ray showed pneumonia. She also correctly omitted enalapril, a recommendation the patient's mother was not made aware of. After asking a nurse, she gave the drug to the patient, which subsequently resulted in his death. Before death, the patient was also moved to a room that, earlier in that day, was occupied by a child of similar age with a do not resuscitate (DNAR) order. Dr Bawa-Garba mistook the patient's identity and did not resuscitate him after he went into cardiac shock.[9]

Dr Bawa-Garba was later charged with gross negligence and manslaughter, while the consultant on call and the nurse faced no charges. Additionally, she was also sentenced to jail for 24 months, which was later changed to a 24-month suspended sentence. The GMC appealed to erase her registration from the UK medical register, to which the Medical Practitioners Tribunal Service (MPTS) appealed. Ultimately, she was struck off the medical register for a year. However, in 2018, the GMC successfully appealed to the court to stop her from practising. It was met with severe criticism from all fronts. After the case was analysed several times, Dr Bawa-Garba was allowed to practice from July 2019 onwards under certain conditions.

Note that despite the conditions of the paediatric department being clearly unfavourable and the trust making numerous changes, it was the junior doctor who was blamed. The short staffing was apparent and had been reported to the hospital administration before the incident happened. Despite several national and international doctors' groups supporting Dr Bawa-Garba, her impeccable records and support from expert paediatricians and the GMC's own tribunal, she had to suffer irrevocable harm, mentally and professionally.[10, 11]

This case points out the gap in the system. Experts agreed that there was no one person to blame when the system itself was working against Dr Bawa-Garba. The NHS, with an overload of patients and clearly not enough resources, needs reforming/more investment if these situations are to be avoided in future.

Nevertheless, the lesson here for juniors is that they must note every detail of their conversations with their supervisor regarding any patient. It is not sufficient to note only that a conversation occurred. Questions asked, concerns had, information relayed, exact responses and instructions regarding treatment should be clearly documented. Even then, these notes may not be accepted in court and it can end up in a 'he said, she said' argument.

STANDARD EXPECTED OF THE JUNIOR DOCTOR

According to the current law, any trainee doctor found to be negligent will be judged by the same standard as an experienced doctor. It does not mean that a junior doctor is expected to have the same level of skills and experience as a senior doctor at all times. Instead, a junior doctor is expected to have the abilities of an average doctor in the same position and will be judged based on the role they are fulfilling. For example, if they perform a surgical procedure, they will be judged by the same standard as a qualified surgeon. If they examine a patient, they will be expected to have a reasonable level of skills to recognise signs and symptoms correctly in line with their professional duty of care. If a doctor does not feel capable of delivering safe care, they should not deliver it; therefore, the excuse of being junior and not knowing enough is invalid.

A common statement made by health care professionals when giving evidence is that they raised concerns about the system many times and these were ignored. The response will be that if you felt the system was unsafe then you should not have been working in it. Clearly this is an impossible situation as you cannot walk away from your role and professional obligations. Recently, following the tragic events at the Countess of Chester Hospital where warnings regarding Lucy Letby were ignored by managers, there may be more focus on managers taking responsibility for not responding to concerns; however, currently there is no such statute. Doctors who raise concerns are still potentially seen as trouble makers even though they should be protected by the Public Interest Disclosure Act from suffering detriment.

The Wilsher v Essex Area Health Authority case is an example of how this issue plays out before the law.[12] The case involved an infant who had been delivered prematurely and was given oxygen by the junior doctor in charge, who accidentally provided too much. Later, the baby developed retinal damage; the junior doctor's actions were determined to be one of the five factors that caused the injury. The final decision was that 'a junior doctor owed the same duty of care as a fully qualified doctor'.

Similarly, in George Andrews v Greater Glasgow Health Board, the defendant junior doctor was held accountable for discharging a patient who came in with suspected melaena secondary to aspirin and later died after developing acute mesenteric ischaemia. The defendant argued that the case was discussed with the consultant in charge. However, the judge ruled that the junior doctor misled the consultant and should have insisted on admitting the patient, as any experienced doctor would do. As the judge mentioned in his ruling, 'It is well known, a learner driver must show the same standard of care as any other driver, and the same applies to junior doctors'.[13]

The Wilsher case is also popular for establishing the law that the 'the Claimant always holds the burden of proving likely causation'. This means that if the subject of legal proceedings is found to have breached their duty of care, the patient/claimant is responsible for proving that the former's actions were the reason or one of the reasons for or a material contribution to the harm.

For junior doctors the best course of action is to be sure of their own competence and skills and not overstretch themselves. When given a responsibility, they should be equipped to handle it. Otherwise, the senior should be notified immediately. As previously stated, historically, trainees took pride in never contacting their seniors and in handling anything that came along. These days, this is not sensible and will invite criticism and increase the risk of harm to patients.

A mistake should be reported to the consultant or immediate senior at once. It is beneficial for all, especially the doctor who made the mistake, that the harm to the patient is as minimal as possible and failure to speedily rectify the error can be deemed to be negligent in itself. Notifying the correct person and the wider team is certain to prevent further damage.[14]

Admittedly, there is a persistent need for a better feedback system in the NHS. Juniors will make mistakes. Accepting this universal truth, intervention methods with personalised, structured feedback systems need to be in place to ensure a safer environment for both patients and trainee doctors.[15]

Junior doctors must ensure that they are continually improving their skills and knowledge when working as health professionals to be able to handle all of the situations they may face in their careers. They might never be fully prepared for all circumstances, but they should provide the standard of care expected from their position as junior doctors.

REFERENCES

1. Shibu, P. K., Subramonian, S., Suresh, M., Vindlacheruvu, M., Cheeroth, S., & Myint, P. K. (2008). Junior doctors' awareness of terminology relating to key medico-legal and ethical principles: A questionnaire survey. *Clinical Medicine*, 8(2), 231.
2. Lewis, P. J., Ashcroft, D. M., Dornan, T., Taylor, D., Wass, V., & Tully, M. P. (2014). Exploring the causes of junior doctors' prescribing mistakes: A qualitative study. *British Journal of Clinical Pharmacology*, 78(2), 310–319.
3. Ryan, C., Ross, S., Davey, P., Duncan, E. M., Fielding, S., Francis, J. J., ... Bond, C. (2013). Junior doctors' perceptions of their self-efficacy in prescribing, their prescribing errors and the possible causes of errors. *British Journal of Clinical Pharmacology*, 76(6), 980–987.
4. Hutchinson, B., Conley, C., Collins, C., Downey, E., Jenkins, J., Sales, L., ... Roades, S. (2021). *Miscommunication among healthcare professionals in the hospital setting: A quality improvement project.* https://scholarworks.moreheadstate.edu/celebration_videos_2021/21.

5. Shaw, N. (2022, February 15). *Doctor gave fatal overdose after miscom-munication partly thanks to masks. WalesOnline.* Retrieved from https://www.walesonline.co.uk/news/uk-news/doctor-gave-fatal-overdose-after-23104136.

6. Hayes, A. J., Pool, R., Roughley, C., Scholes, S., Sharifi, L., Woodside, R., ... Singleton, L. (2018). Communication and miscommunication: Handover between junior doctors. *Reinvention: An International Journal of Undergraduate Research*, 11(1). https://warwick.ac.uk/fac/cross_fac/iatl/reinvention/archive/volume5issue1/hayes

7. O'Connor, P., O'Dea, A., Lydon, S., Offiah, G., Scott, J., Flannery, A., ... Byrne, D. (2016). A mixed-methods study of the causes and impact of poor teamwork between junior doctors and nurses. *International Journal for Quality in Health Care*, 28(3), 339–345.

8. Voigt, P., & Von dem Bussche, A. (2017). The EU General Data Protection Regulation (GDPR). A practical guide. *Springer, Cham International Publishing*, 10(3152676), 10–5555.

9. Nicholl, D. (2018). *Bawa-Garba case: GMC failed in its job as a regulator. British Medical Journal*, https://doi.org/10.1136/bmj.k4111.

10. Rimmer, A. (2018). 'We would employ Hadiza Bawa-Garba,' say 159 paediatricians. *British Medical Journal*, 361. https://doi.org/10.1136/bmj.k2393.

11. McCartney, M. (2018). Margaret McCartney: Clinical errors need a systemic response. *British Medical Journal*, 360. https://doi.org/10.1136/bmj.k812.

12. Wilsher v Essex Area Health Authority. (2013, November). *Law teacher.* Retrieved from https://www.lawteacher.net/cases/wilsher-v-essex-area-health-authority.php?vref=1.

13. Dyer, C. (2019). Junior doctor was negligent in not admitting patient who later died, judge rules. *British Medical Journal*, 365. https://doi.org/10.1136/bmj.l1576.

14. Millwood, S. (2014). Developing a platform for learning from mistakes: Changing the culture of patient safety amongst junior doctors. *BMJ Open Quality*, 3(1), u203658–w2114.

15. Green, W., Shahzad, M. W., Wood, S., Martinez Martinez, M., Baines, A., Navid, A., ... Patel, R. (2020). Improving junior doctor medicine prescribing and patient safety: An intervention using personalised, structured, video-enhanced feedback and deliberate practice. *British Journal of Clinical Pharmacology*, 86(11), 2234–2246.

11

Remote consultations and medicolegal implications

With the outbreak of the highly contagious coronavirus 2019, the entire world was forced to go into lockdown. While medical organisations remained open, there were fundamental risks and challenges in seeing patients. The most obvious solution was to change key delivery methods to digital, something that many felt was long overdue. Remote consultations became a primary mode of continuing care, as patients were not allowed to travel or leave their homes during this period. Telemedicine was one such process that played a significant role in making health care reachable and convenient for both doctors and patients.

Telemedicine in the UK has been mostly welcomed, although some patients still wish for more face-to-face appointments. According to a news article published in the *New York Times*, telemedicine has brought 10 years' worth of change in a few weeks.[1]

The advantage of telemedicine or digital medical services is obvious. It is convenient, time saving (at least for the patients) and flexible. However, from a medicolegal point of view, telemedicine is filled with potential medicolegal pitfalls and may be prone to leaving clinicians open to allegations of substandard care.

Remote consultations are not the gold standard of care. Nothing can replace seeing a patient in the flesh and being able to examine them with the practitioner's own eyes and hands. Telemedicine is a compromise with significant benefits but also significant downsides. The courts have not yet formulated definitive guidance as to what standard of care should be expected from a teleconsultation versus a face-to-face consultation and whether there will be any leeway or lower acceptable standard taking into account the inherent weakness of the remote consultation format. At the moment, the standard is the same for remote and face-to-face consultations. Misdiagnosing patients is possible even when we see them in the flesh; thus, the risks of teleconsultation must inevitably be higher.

With time, the Bolam/Bolitho tests may adapt, and the standard of care may be that of a reasonably competent doctor undertaking a telemedicine consultation. However, at present, that is not the case, which makes the need for caution

DOI: 10.1201/9781003179351-14

and diligence when diagnosing and treating patients remotely all the more important.

Inevitable, and naturally, if harm occurs due to a misdiagnosis made via a remote consultation then the patient will assert that it would not have occurred had they been seen 'properly'.

The GMC has some specific guidance on remote consultations.[2] They provide a diagram to help decision making as to whether a remote consultation is appropriate as indicated here.

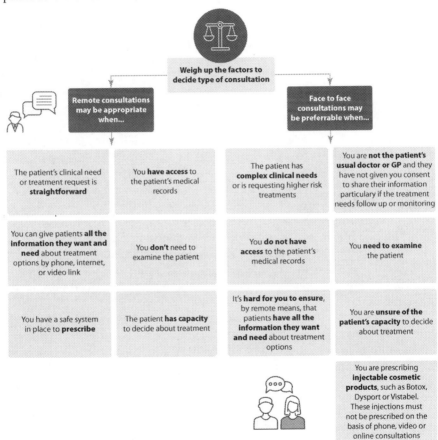

When a remote consultation is undertaken:

- *Record keeping*: Make sure you take detailed notes during the consultation because you will be held liable and judged by the same standard as a regular consultation.
- *Limitations*: It is important that the patient is aware of the limitations of a remote consultation. If you feel that a remote consultation is not adequate to assess the patient, make it clear to them and arrange for them to be seen. Be aware of the limitations yourself and ask yourself if you can be confident of a

diagnosis without an examination. How will your conduct be viewed if you are incorrect?

- *Consent*: Obtaining consent is vital for all consultations, even in telemedicine. Inform the patient that the conversation is being recorded and that everything they say is protected by doctor–patient confidentiality. They should also know that they have the right to seek or not seek treatment. Be aware that the consultation may be recorded at the patient's side and used as evidence if harm occurs due to your decisions.

- *Communication*: Communication is the key to telemedicine. Introduce yourself and explain the nature of the consultation. Obviously, you have to rely on the patient to provide a full and accurate description of their illness. Take your time and establish a relationship of trust with the patient before asking details about their symptoms. The patient will be able to provide quite accurate information if they are relaxed. Look directly at the camera and not the screen to maintain eye contact. For many older patients, telecommunication is difficult and exhausting. Keep that in mind while consulting.

- *Sticking to the basics*: Telemedicine or video consulting is still a consultation, and the same principles apply. This means taking the patient's medical history, medication history, social history and family history. The clinical examination is more challenging. If the consultation is via video, then it is possible to be shown a rash, for example; however, a proper examination is not possible. Asking the patient to describe their symptoms as clearly as possible is vital, and they can self-examine to some degree. Clearly, this is not ideal, and if an error occurs, it may be criticised.

- *Defence*: Whether the patient needs a face-to-face consultation depends on the doctor's medical judgement. However, in case of any negative outcome, the doctor must be able to defend their decision with sound logic. Hence, all conversations must be recorded, and thorough questions must be asked. You may want to take more time during a teleconsultation for the sake of an accurate diagnosis. When things go wrong, patients may be less forgiving. Not all patients want a teleconsultation: 'I wanted to see a GP but could not get an appointment. Instead, she just phoned me. No wonder she got it wrong'.

- *Past documentation*: Make sure that you have access to the patient's previous clinical information, medical records, investigations, radiology reports, etc. Any alteration to the previous treatment should be explained in the records. Sometimes, telemedicine may be carried out without any previous records. This is fraught with risk, and caution should be exercised.

- *Safety netting*: Teleconsultation can be severely restrictive. When finishing the consultation, always have a safety net in place. Give the patient proper instructions on how to contact you or emergency services if their situation deteriorates. They should also be notified of which signs to look for (e.g. sudden and severe vomiting after a fall) and when to seek further attention. This should all be clearly documented in the clinical record.

WHEN TO REQUEST A FACE-TO-FACE CONSULTATION

- If you feel that the patient is suffering from a complex clinical situation.
- If the patient has a chronic condition that is paining them, and you are not their usual doctor.
- If you do not have adequate documents on the patient's previous condition or you cannot communicate with the patient clearly.
- If you are unsure about the patient's mental capability of consenting to treatment.
- If repeated teleconsultations are failing to remedy the issue, then consider bringing the patient in for review to ensure you are not missing anything. If there is an issue then it will look bad if the patient can state 'I had five video consultations but the doctor refused to see me face-to-face'.

Telemedicine comes with inherent risks, such as misdiagnosis and failure to identify, treat or provide adequate care to the patient. However, it is immensely helpful, and it will inevitably remain even after the pandemic is contained. We need to adapt and work with it while protecting ourselves and patients. You cannot examine a patient properly via telemedicine, and it is vital that you acknowledge the limitations yourself and relay those to the patient.

At present, you will be judged as if you physically examined the patient, and so, it is vital that caution is exercised. The Royal College of General Practitioners and other bodies have advice as to how to handle remote consultations. It is important that you familiarise yourself with this advice and adhere to it.

Only time will tell whether there is leniency and 'the benefit of the doubt' offered to doctors and health care professionals who misdiagnose/mismanage patients who are solely treated by remote means.

REFERENCES

1. Mueller, B. (2020). Telemedicine arrives in the UK: '10 years of change in one week'. *New York Times*.
2. Remote Consultations. (2022). *General Medical Council*. Retrieved from https://www.gmc-uk.org/ethical-guidance/ethical-hub/remote-consultations.

12

Locums

Locums have been and will always be a part of the health care in the NHS. Locums are temporary medical staff who fill gaps in permanent medical rotas by providing short-term cover for planned and unplanned absences. The majority of locum doctors are employed by specialist agencies offering doctors to fill shifts or vacancies on a temporary basis, usually for durations ranging from half a day to a few weeks.

Temporary staff are also used widely in nursing and other health care settings with the use of agency or bank staff, and similar issues can apply to them.

Although important for delivering safe care, there is a perceived concern about the quality of care being delivered by locums. Little evidence suggests that locums as a group are less safe than permanent doctors, but there are some factors that may lead to poorer performance. These include a lack of familiarity with local systems, such as different drug formularies and procedures, a lack of familiarity with colleagues, lower levels of integration into the team and difficulties with handovers between shifts. In addition, locums may have no contractual responsibility to address any substandard performance on their part, which would otherwise be addressed through appraisal or disciplinary procedures if they were permanent staff members. This creates a concern in many employers as well.

Despite this perception, no definitive evidence or study shows that the work of a locum doctor is substandard to a contracted doctor. In fact, many doctors work both in fixed positions and as locums in their free time. Thus, there is very little difference in the actual skill. The difficulties are mostly systemic and due to unfamiliarity with local working practices and logistics.

There is also the tendency for more media attention to clinical errors by locums as it is of more interest to the general public and therefore perceptions may be altered.

A solution lies in improving the support systems available for locums. This can be achieved by providing appropriate induction programmes, including training on local policies and procedures, and introducing clear systems for reporting incidents, locally and nationally.

DOI: 10.1201/9781003179351-15

LOCUMS AND THE CLINICAL NEGLIGENCE SCHEME FOR TRUSTS

All doctors working in the UK performing NHS-commissioned work are covered by an indemnity scheme starting from 2019. The Clinical Negligence Scheme for Trusts (CNST) covers all doctors commissioned by the NHS.[1] These include locums and out-of-hours services, as well as regular salaried doctors. Anyone working with clinics associated with the NHS, urgent care services, social care or out-of-hours services is covered by the CNST or, for GPs, the Clinical Negligence Scheme for General Practice (CNSGP).

THE PITFALLS AND DIFFICULTIES OF BEING A LOCUM

In 2008, a locum doctor from Germany, Dr U, was covering an out-of-hours shift in the UK at a PCT. He was found guilty of negligence when he accidentally overdosed a patient with 100 mg of diamorphine. While it appeared to be a straightforward case of severely substandard care, some mitigating circumstances were highlighted by the investigation. The doctor was not prepared adequately for his shift. He had received an induction by the local GP, but no hands-on demonstration was given regarding the palliative care box that contained several ampules, including 10 mg and 100 mg of diamorphine. The coroner mentioned in his report that it was not Dr U's intention to kill the patient and that the death was accidental. Despite these excuses, the level of care was unacceptable, and the doctor was guilty of negligence. Dr U was given a 9-month suspended sentence in Germany and was struck off by the GMC.[2] It is of interest that the same firm had two other diamorphine overdose incidents prior to this one and still had not prepared the doctors accordingly or removed the 100 mg ampules. The doctor who gave the locum the induction also raised concerns over the under-preparedness of the locum doctor, but this was only read 2 days after the patient had died.

This case is one of many that shed light on several hidden factors a locum doctor needs to be aware of. Here are some common pitfalls and tips on how to avoid them:

- *Not being familiar with the medication in the hospital region the doctor is working in*: This can be a common source of error and potential harm. Generic names for drugs should always be used if possible. However, brand names can sometimes be used, which can lead to confusion. Not being familiar with packaging sizes and dosage can easily lead to the administration of lethal doses.

- *Problems occurring with locum doctors not following local protocols and practices*: A study on clinical support and interprofessional interactions showed that most nurses felt that locum doctors took more time to respond to referrals on clinical support calls because they were not aware of the context.[3] According to another small study, the locum anaesthetists often did not follow the same steps (e.g. not doing the site check) as the in-house anaesthetists. If errors occur, then the most obvious standard to which a doctor's performance will be compared will be the local protocols. Failure to adhere to them is very hard to defend.

- *Supervision and support*: Locum doctors are usually unaware of the local systems that exist in a practice or hospital setting. They may be unaware of the local lines of communication and who to call when they need advice. There may be a tendency not to bother fellow doctors, and there may even be hostility from colleagues who do not want to be 'troubled by the locum'. Such sentiment undermines and is detrimental to all within the department. Permanent clinicians have a vested interest in supporting locums, as locums will move away while the local doctors will be left to pick up the pieces of error and harm.

Practice can vary massively between countries, and therefore it is particularly important to support foreign doctors working for the first time in the NHS.

Adequate induction and support can allay many of the problems the locum doctor faces. It is in the best interests of the employing organisation and their clinical colleagues to ensure that locums have all the education and support they need. The whole team needs to engage to prevent the risk of error and harm.

WHO TAKES RESPONSIBILITY?

According to Ferguson and Walshe, the factors that influence the quality and safety of locum doctors' treatments have very little to do with the doctors themselves and more with the 'organisations who use locums and the ways in which they (locum) are deployed and supported'.[4] Failure to prepare the doctor, rushing them to an emergency condition with no guidelines, not providing a proper induction and failing to provide adequate instructions ultimately lead to accidents, errors and harm that may result in complaints and/or litigation. Ferguson and Walshe concluded that 'the quality and safety of locum practice is fundamentally shaped by the organisational context in which they work'.

Even in the presence of mitigating organisational circumstances or evidenced inadequate induction, the standard that the locum doctor needs to meet is the same as that of any other doctor. As a patient being treated by that individual it makes sense and is right.

Locum doctors should make every effort to follow local protocols, and if they are unsure, they should ask. For their part, organisations and clinical colleagues should make every effort to ensure that locum doctors have this support in place.

Lastly, there may be a perception that the locum doctor is somehow inferior to the regular doctor. Patients can often feel aggrieved that they 'saw the locum', and they may be less forgiving of any errors that may occur. Permanent staff may not support the locum, which can propagate issues and escalate complaints, thus being detrimental to everyone involved.

REFERENCES

1. https://resolution.nhs.uk/services/claims-management/clinical-schemes/clinical-negligence-scheme-for-trusts/.
2. BMJ. (2010). 341:c3869.
3. Young, S, K., Young, T, K. (2016). Assessing clinical support and inter-professional interactions among front-line primary care providers in remote communities in northern Canada: A pilot study. *International Journal of Circumpolar Health*, 75: 10.3402.
4. Ferguson, J., Walshe, K. (2019). The quality and safety of locum doctors: A narrative review. *Journal of the Royal Society of Medicine*, 112(11), 462–471. doi:10.1177/0141076819877539.

SECTION 4

Dealing with complaints

13

The National Health Service complaints process

COMPLAINTS TO THE NHS

Written complaints about NHS services have more than doubled between 2005/2006 and 2017/2018. In 2005/2006, there were 95,047 complaints or 1,827 a week, compared with 208,626 or 4,017 a week in 2017/2018. GP practices received approximately 1 written complaint for every 4,200 appointments in 2018/2019, based on data from NHS digital.[1] The factors that influence the number of complaints include the ability of local organisations to resolve issues when they first arise and patient awareness of the Patients Advice Service (PALs).

THE NATIONAL HEALTH SERVICE COMPLAINTS REGULATIONS

Any doctor practising within the NHS must know how to deal with complaints and how to negotiate the NHS complaints procedure. As clinicians, it can be difficult to think like a patient. Things that seem very obvious to a doctor may not be to a patient without any clinical background and experience. On the other hand, arguments that seem plausible to a patient may seem outrageous to a doctor. For example, a patient may be concerned about eye issues after a tooth extraction when there is no physiological or pathological link between them.

No matter how weak a complaint or how unreasonable an assertion may seem, the patient deserves full attention from the practice or organisation to try and address their issues. Closing complaints too quickly, reacting defensively or dismissing a complaint outright without any investigation can escalate the situation unnecessarily, often ultimately resulting in litigation. Many patients are aware of numerous adverts for no-win no-fee services who will assist with clinical negligence claims.

The cost, stress, time and efforts will be far higher and more painful to resolve through litigation than solving a simple complaint early on. Therefore, dealing with complaints is a skill worth learning.

The regulations are slightly different between England and the devolved nations, and it is important to be familiar with the regulations, wherever we work. The general principles, however, are universal.

The National Health Service Complaints Regulations were formulated in 2009 to better understand and respond to patients' complaints.[2] The document has been upgraded and added to in the following years.[3] As the most suited people to handle complaints are the organisations the complaints are filed against, the NHS regulations make sure that all health service providers and health professionals are legally, contractually and professionally obligated to provide the ideal place to manage a patient's complaint.

Furthermore, an obligation to fully cooperate and facilitate the process has been enshrined.

The regulations impose strict requirements for every practice/hospital. These are the key elements of the regulations. An extensive list includes requirements to make the process of filing and dealing with complaints easy for everyone.

'The practice must have arrangements in place to handle complaints efficiently, investigating them properly and delivering a timely and appropriate response. It must make information about these arrangements available to the public'. Thus, NHS practices/hospitals have a duty to have services specifically in place to handle complaints and make the information about them clearly available for patients.

Organisations are required to ensure the proper and fair handling of complaints by appointing one person as the 'responsible person' who takes overarching responsibility for them. Additionally, they are responsible for ensuring that the teaching or learning points from the complaints are being practised. There should also be a designated complaints manager who is responsible for managing all the complaints coming into the practice or organisation. Both of these roles can be fulfilled by the same person.

According to the complaints regulations, anyone affected by decisions, actions and omissions or any person acting as a representative can file a complaint.

However, any third party needs to be proven to be working in the best interest of the patient.

The PHSO's Principles of Good Complaint Handling mentions six key principles that are central to good complaints handling.[4] The ombudsman expects to see these applied to complaints handled by all public bodies, including NHS bodies and organisations providing NHS services.

- Getting it right
- Being customer focused
- Being open and accountable
- Acting fairly and proportionately
- Putting things right
- Seeking continuous improvement

Stage one of the NHS complaints procedure involves resolving complaints at the local level. In most instances, that is the GP practice or hospital concerned. The NHS complaints procedure emphasises resolving complaints as quickly as possible and, ideally, locally. Speed, sympathy, willingness to listen and effective, considerate communication are often all that are needed.

Timing is important when dealing with complaints. If an oral complaint is handled with the patient successfully within one working day, it does not even fall within the scope of the regulations. If this cannot be achieved, both written and oral complaints need to be acknowledged within 3 working days.

When acknowledging, the practice or doctor should not acknowledge any fault or make any inference as to the validity of the complaint, but they can accept the fact that there is a complaint. In the acknowledgement, it is good practice to suggest a place or time for a phone call when the details of the case can be discussed and information gathered. The practice or organisation then investigates the complaint once all the relevant information is gathered.

It is unlikely that a hospital doctor will write the response, but they need to provide an account of what happened to help the complaints manager write a response. They may also be asked to discuss the complaint, which may include meeting with the complainant.

It is vital that complainants are kept informed of the process and timescales involved. The responsible body should keep a record of the complaints, record any lessons learnt, consider and monitor complaints as part of its clinical governance procedures and provide an annual report that should be available on request. Primary care providers should also send a report to the commissioning body.

At every level, it is important that records are kept of what actions are taken in response to complaints, and these must be kept separate from patients' records. Keeping careful records will help manage complaints and also provide evidence of effective complaint handling if a complaint is reviewed by the ombudsman.

REFERENCES

1. Tabner, A., Tilbury, N., Jones, M., Fakis, A., Evans, N., Johnson, G. (2022). Trends in emergency department litigation within the NHS: A retrospective database analysis. *Medico-Legal Journal*, 90(1), 5–12. doi:10.1177/00258172211057000.
2. Local Authority Social Services and National Health Service Complaints (England) Regulations. (2009). https://www.legislation.gov.uk/uksi/2009/309/contents/made.
3. https://www.england.nhs.uk/publication/nhs-england-complaints-policy/.
4. Nason, S. (2020). European principles of good administration and UK administrative justice. *European Public Law*, 26(2).

14

Independent sector complaints processes

Private health care organisations and hospitals are a large part of health care services in the UK. While private hospitals are not required to abide by the same laws and regulations imposed on NHS hospitals, a similar standard of care is expected, and most hospitals have a code or framework in place that ensures seamless complaint management.

The ISCAS Code of Practice for Complaints Management (ISCAS Code) was established to provide similar support and guidelines as the NHS for privately owned hospitals and organisations in dealing with complaints. The ISCAS Code applies to all complaints by patients who are dissatisfied with services provided by independent health care providers (IHPs). These IHPs include hospitals and clinics that provide services paid for directly by the patient or an insurance scheme. In some instances, it may also include private patient units in NHS hospitals, where they are subscribers to the ISCAS.

The ISCAS Code sets out the standards that all subscribing IHPs are expected to follow when dealing with complaints about their services. It is designed to ensure that patients/customers receive a fair response when things go wrong. Subscribing IHPs agree to abide by the code. If an IHP breaks the code, the ISCAS does not have any statutory power to enforce it; however, actions will be taken against the organisation, including termination of the subscription.

The ISCAS functions are based on a similar framework to that of the NHS's, namely the PHSO's Principles of Good Complaint Handling (2009). Like governmental organisations, the independent sector handles complaints in several steps, depending on severity and failure to resolve. The code does not cover unlawful acts, criminal acts, financial disputes, clinical negligence, mental health act issues, NHS patients and private medical insurance products. Complaints regarding these should go to the appropriate authority (e.g. the police or the court). Only complaints regarding service and treatment can be processed through the ISCAS.

DOI: 10.1201/9781003179351-18

ISCAS-mediated steps are specific and involve the health care professional. They include:

- *Local resolution*: When a patient or anyone on their behalf complains about a hospital or practice, the first step is to try and resolve it locally. The ISCAS requires that the process of complaint submission should be clear and concise and that all patients should have access to help if needed, such as to overcome a language barrier or disability. Upon receiving the complaint, the IHP is required to consider and investigate it. If an independent investigation is needed, the IHP bears the cost for it. A written acknowledgement must be sent to the complainant within 3 days and a full response to the complaint within 20 working days.

- *Complaint review*: If the complaint is not resolved locally or the patient is not satisfied with the measures taken, they may want to take it to the next level. At the next stage, the complaint, along with all documentation, is analysed and reviewed. Stage two may need face-to-face meetings and discussions with the involved staff. The timing deadline of 3 and 20 days applies to this stage as well.

- *Independent external adjudication*: This last stage is only undertaken when the complaint cannot be managed by the IHPs. This step is mediated by the ISCAS. An adjudicator will oversee handling the documentation and mediation.

The Independent External Adjudication (IEA) is a public body that handles complaints against IHPs. It is important to note that the IEA does not represent the health care provider or the patient. Their responsibility is only to investigate the complaint, mediate discussions between the parties and suggest whether an expert needs to be hired to ascertain whether a health care provider has acted within their rights and responsibilities in accordance with relevant laws.

Ultimately, the adjudication decision is final. For health care professionals, the prime responsibility is to comply with the ISCAS and provide any documents and records needed.

15

Duty of candour

A duty of candour is owed to every patient under a health care professional's care. Health care professionals have an obligation to inform their patients about any events that may result in harm and provide all information about their treatment or any mistakes that may have happened. This is a part of the larger duty of providers to be honest with their patients. Candour is expected of doctors and helps to build rapport between patient and provider, which can help improve patient satisfaction and treatment adherence. The courts will look upon attempts to deceive or withhold information very poorly. Nevertheless, some downsides to candour can be expected.

The first potential but unavoidable harm caused by candour is that patients will often assume lack of expertise or skill on the health care professional or doctor's part. Unavoidable developments or idiopathic conditions are also often blamed on the doctor, and if errors are detailed in a letter in black and white, there is an all too human desire for recompense and compensation. The numerous no-win no-fee negligence solicitor firms make it all too easy to launch a claim. On the one hand, patients should be allowed to seek recompense for harm, but on the other hand, frivolous unjustified claims can incur significant costs and harm to doctors related to the stress and distress of handling the complaint.

Without a doubt patients deserve justice and recompense if they have come to avoidable harm and claimants' solicitor firms undertake an invaluable role in assisting patients in getting what they deserve.

Patients or families often wish to file claims against the doctor or health care facility when their loved one's health takes a bad turn. Many clinical negligence allegations are made based on frustration and anger.

The situation only gets worse when a definite mistake has been made, which has been identified by an internal investigation, and harm has occurred. Considering the rates of litigation, many providers are uncomfortable with apologising because they fear that it will be used against them as an admission of guilt. As we have discussed before, this is not true.

The duty of candour is inviolate and must be practised. It is the right of any patient to be fully informed regarding their care and the integrity of their health and body. All information, whether good or bad, must be relayed to the patient.

 DOI: 10.1201/9781003179351-19

Often, the way this communication is undertaken will have an impact on what transpires thereafter.

The GMC offers excellent guidance as to what our duty of candour entails.[6] It states that:

> Every healthcare professional must be open and honest with patients when something that goes wrong with their treatment or care causes, or has the potential to cause, harm or distress. This means that healthcare professionals must:
>
> - tell the patient (or, where appropriate, the patient's advocate, carer or family) when something has gone wrong
> - apologise to the patient (or, where appropriate, the patient's advocate, carer or family)
> - offer an appropriate remedy or support to put matters right (if possible) explain fully to the patient (or, where appropriate, the patient's advocate, carer or family) the short- and long-term effects of what has happened.

Duty of candour letters will inevitably trigger litigation, but their very nature is sometimes misinterpreted. Trusts actively seek to find harm and errors, learn from them and put in place measures to prevent them happening again. They are designed to be critical of current practice to allow us to evolve and change practice going forwards to protect patients. Acknowledgement of harm and suggestions for change are not always the same as admitting negligent treatment, and the concern is that duty of candour letters and responses to complaints are used as a 'stick to beat the clinician with'.

Health care professionals must also be open and honest with their colleagues, employers and relevant organisations and take part in reviews and investigations when requested. They must also be open and honest with their regulators, raising concerns where appropriate. They must support and encourage each other to be open and honest and not stop someone from raising concerns.

All health care professionals have a duty of candour – a professional responsibility to be honest with patients when things go wrong. This is described in The professional duty of candour,[1] which introduces this guidance and forms part of a joint statement from eight regulators of health care professionals in the UK.

In addition to the individual's obligations, organisations have a duty of candour to support their staff to report adverse incidents and to be open and honest with patients if something goes wrong with their care.

Most patients simply wish for an apology, to understand what went wrong and assurance that it will not happen to anyone again.

REFERENCE

1. General Medical Council. The Professional Duty of Candour. https://www
   .gmc-uk.org/professional-standards/professional-standards-for-doctors
   /candour---openness-and-honesty-when-things-go-wrong/the-profes-
   sional-duty-of-candour.

16

Responding to the complaint

The tone of your response needs to be professional, measured and sympathetic. Be careful about disclosing any patient information or third-party data without explicit permission.

There are time constraints, and you should not introduce undue delay. However, it is also important to take your time and think about your response carefully before submitting it. Do not let your emotion cloud your response, and leave it overnight before sending it. Often the response will be sent to your manager or complaints handling team first, but bear in mind that it may be sent to the patient at some stage. More importantly remember that it will inevitably be disclosed to the patient's legal team if litigation ensues.

The complaint may be about you, or it may relate to the conduct of your team or colleagues. The main purpose of the complaints procedure is to address the complainant's concerns, resolve the complaint and help you identify any changes needed to improve your practice.

A thorough and detailed first response should help minimise the risk of the complainant asking for clarification and the risk of any further escalation of the complaint or even litigation. Put your case forward in a sensible and logical way. The information in your response will be included in the correspondence with the patient but will not be copied to the patient in its entirety at the first stage. You have a duty to the patient to assist them, a duty to learn from the complaint and adapt your/your team's future practice if appropriate and a duty to your organisation and the NHS as a whole.

Remember that the letter you/your practice/your trust send to the patient will potentially be sent to a clinical negligence lawyer and may be available to the court if a claim is made. If a complaint is made to a primary care organisation rather than to a GP practice, the doctor(s)/health care professionals involved should be fully consulted and have the opportunity to provide statements about their involvement. The organisation might also seek independent expert advice on the complaint's clinical aspects. In secondary care, a written response can be sent from the chief executive or a responsible person on their behalf.

Include a factual chronology of events, which can be from the medical record or your recollections. It is acceptable to quote from memory, but if you cannot

DOI: 10.1201/9781003179351-20

remember the details of the case, you may say what your 'usual' or 'normal' practice would have been in those circumstances. This response does not need to be as detailed as that provided if the case does progress to formal litigation, but it is important to do the first step correctly, as all future evidence will be built upon it. Changing your position/statement later can be used against you, so be consistent and be honest.

Try and address each point raised by the complainant, including your opinion of what happened. Many complaints come from misunderstandings, and a detailed description of the reasoning behind any management decision can help, although care should be taken to avoid medical terms and jargon.

Exercise caution when commenting on the conduct of a fellow clinician or colleague, unless they are under your direct supervision. It is entirely reasonable to say sorry where appropriate. You are a health care provider, and, if a patient under your care has to complain about the care they receive, then you have failed them to some degree, even if there is no fault at all.

Section 2 of the Compensation Act 2006 states that 'an apology, an offer of treatment or other redress, shall not of itself amount to an admission of negligence or breach of statutory duty'.[1] The response should include what you have done or intend to do to remedy the concerns identified and make sure the problem does not happen again. If you feel that you have not done anything wrong, then it is reasonable to say so. However, you must not come across as arrogant or dismissive of the complainant's concerns.

Once the investigation is completed, the response letter can be sent, which answers each facet of the complaint, explains how it has been investigated, details what action will be taken as a result and clearly advises that the complainant can take the case to the ombudsman if they are still dissatisfied. If the initial complaint is non-serious in nature, often, a written apology will suffice.

Other times, a more formal approach is needed. However, it must be clear that all efforts were made when handling the complaint, and appropriate measures were taken without discrimination.

Some complaints cannot be handled by the organisation being complained about. The patient may want to complain through other organisations if they feel it necessary. For example, if a patient is unhappy with the response to a complaint against a GP practice, they can escalate the complaint to the primary care trust (PCT). The PCT can take up the complaint, handle the case and keep both the practice and the patient updated regarding the progress and final outcome of the investigation.

When all attempts have failed to solve the case locally and the first stage of the NHS complaints procedure has failed, the complainant can refer their complaint to the Parliamentary and Health Service Ombudsman (PHSO) for investigation. This is stage two of the procedure.

The ombudsman can also consider grievances about the administration of the complaints procedure itself. Complaints should normally be referred to the ombudsman within 12 months of when the complainant first knew about the issue. The ombudsman has discretion to investigate complaints outside this time frame if they deem it appropriate.

The ombudsman considers each case on its merits and can decide whether to investigate a complaint. This highlights the need for a thorough investigation and response at stage one. The ombudsman is required to consider a complaint only when injustice or hardship arises from failure in a service, failure to provide a service or maladministration. If it decides not to investigate a complaint, the ombudsman's office will write to the complainant to explain why.

If deemed appropriate, the ombudsman may obtain independent professional advice with the aid of specialist assessors for clinical issues. The ombudsman then shares a confidential report containing provisional views, with the complainant and subject of the complaint providing a further opportunity to clarify issues. If a complaint gets to the stage where the ombudsman is involved, it is sensible to involve your indemnity provider.

ONLINE COMPLAINTS

Online complaints or negative website comments/reviews can be equally or potentially even more mentally taxing than in-person complaints. This can be extremely upsetting for the doctor concerned, particularly if they feel that their treatment has been unfairly criticised. It is very public, with no validation or chance to challenge assertions. Such negative comments can adversely affect a health care professional's career, and at present, there appears to be little regulation. The best way to deal with this kind of situation is to take appropriate action as soon as possible.

Below are a few steps you can take if you are made aware of a negative online review about you or your practice:

- Find out what the complaint is about and whether the negative online comment refers to you or your practice.

- Stop and take stock of the situation. Before doing anything else, it is important to read the review carefully and consider whether it is fair or not. If you believe that it is not, then ask yourself what you can do about it. Take your time to think about what was said and whether it needs addressing. Remember that everyone is entitled to their opinion and that not all reviews need to be answered. If you feel that a response is necessary, consult any relevant guidance from the organisation(s) concerned (e.g. the GMC). Even though no real checks are in place to prevent patients from attacking professionals in the public domain, the converse is not true; an attack on a patient in response to online criticism may result in a complaint against you.

- Do not take it personally and do not get angry. It is natural for anyone who believes that they have been unfairly criticised to want to defend themselves, but this is not always in your best interest. You should avoid posting any comments on the site where the review appears, as these are unlikely to help improve your reputation and are likely to make matters worse.

- If you have professional indemnity insurance, discuss the matter with your insurer and ask for advice.

- Negative online reviews can be the result of ill feelings, but they may also reflect a misunderstanding that can easily be rectified. Thus, it is important to establish the reason for any negative review.

- If appropriate, apologise for any mistake or oversight on your part and offer a solution that addresses the reviewer's concerns. This may be as simple as phoning them to discuss their treatment or offering a follow-up. If you feel that the complaint has been resolved, you may ask the patient to take down their original review and replace it with a positive one. Remember that other patients will read the comments and may be able to make their own judgements as to how unreasonable they are. A compassionate and understanding response putting your side of the situation across will look much better than a dismissive or aggressive reply.

- If you feel the comment is not appropriate, you can always ask the website to take it down. In official websites such as NHS Choice, you can report an unhelpful or abusive post so that it can be removed or amended. Without that, there is very little recourse, unfortunately. It is best to scrutinise the terms of the website where the negative comments lie and see whether there is a process to get such comments removed.

If you seek to remove a comment from the NHS Choice website, you will need to state the name of the complainant, your email address, URL for the comment, why it is inaccurate or defamatory, what the comment is implying, a description of the parts of the comment that go against established facts and a confirmation that you do not know the complainant personally. This will be reviewed, and action may be taken. If no action is taken, then legal action can be taken for defamation. To claim for defamation, there has to be evidence of harm or loss. If you are contemplating this, then evidence is vital to show that the comment has been detrimental to you and you have suffered loss. Sadly, hurt feelings are not considered loss.

GENERAL RULES TO FOLLOW

Try to pre-empt and de-escalate

We all know when a complaint is coming. There are typically three scenarios that occur:

- Something unavoidably goes wrong with the care of a patient, and the patient is not happy. In this scenario, the complaint is entirely avoidable with appropriate care and communication. Engage with the patient. Explain what happened and why it was unavoidable. Help them understand that there was nothing else that could have been done and that you are sorry for the harm that has occurred to them, whether physical or mental.

- Something avoidably goes wrong with the care of a patient, and the patient is not happy. Again, a complaint is not inevitable. Most patients understand the pressures that the health service operates under. Explain what happened and empathise with their predicament. Explain what should have happened and how you have made changes to processes/systems/training to avoid a similar circumstance.

- Nothing goes wrong, but the patient had unrealistic expectations. Sadly, this is happening more frequently. Nevertheless, with appropriate, early and empathetic communication, complaints can be avoided. Engage early with such patients and explain what happened and why this was normal.

We all want to deliver great care, but we may not always bond with each patient we treat. That has no bearing on the level of care we must deliver.

It is human nature to try and avoid confrontations or difficult circumstances. These confrontations can be with patients who have run into avoidable harm or 'difficult' patients. We need to actively run towards rather than away from such patients. Meet with them with or without a neutral chaperone. Often, a senior staff member, such as a senior nurse sitting in on the consultation, may help diffuse a situation and satisfy patients that we do care and are taking them seriously.

Do not take complaints personally

This may be impossible to avoid, but you must try. We all work hard to do the best for our patients, and it can be a real hit to face a complaint when we have genuinely done our best. If you have not done your best, then you are obliged to learn from the complaint and improve. Set emotions aside and do not let anger rule. Be analytical but compassionate. Do not allow your frustration to be reflected in your formal response or any interactions with the patient. Remember other patients will see it and an emotional, aggressive or confrontational response will not inspire confidence from other potential patients.

Fully cooperate

Over and above your professional obligations to cooperate with complaints investigations, it is truly in your interest to engage with the management and investigation to either remedy the situation or put forward a strong preliminary defence for your actions. Meet with the investigators, scrutinise the clinical record, present any evidence you find, suggest how things could have been done better and acknowledge any weaknesses you find. Recommend improvements so that these can be relayed to the patient. If the patient realises that you take them seriously and you demonstrate a true conviction to learn and avoid future errors, they can be placated and feel vindicated.

Do not stick your head in the sand. Complaints will not disappear if you ignore them. Add them as a to-do list item to deal with.

Keep records of everything

When things are not going to plan or when a patient appears frustrated or angry, then documentation becomes even more important. Remember that an investigator will be scrutinising notes and documents.

Be professional

As professionals, we will face complaints. Maintain professionalism at all times. Deal with the complaint as another part of your professional duties, just as you would handle any part of the work you do.

Apologise when appropriate

Apologising does not mean accepting blame or responsibility. It is simply a statement of regret for what happened. It is not necessarily a concession that an incident was preventable or foreseeable. An apology can be healing for the patient.

The term 'sorry' may be used in a number of ways, such as:

- I am sorry this happened to you.
- I am sorry you are unhappy about what happened.
- I am sorry I upset you/caused you distress.
- I am sorry that what happened to you was caused by something I did/did not do.

Complaints can be handled well or badly and may escalate if handled inappropriately. If handled badly, they can result in the rapid polarisation of positions, which puts the patient and organisation/health care professional at loggerheads. Emotions can become inflamed, making a resolution challenging to achieve.

Complaints are a fact of professional life and need to be addressed properly. This means putting the complainant first and ensuring that they receive an explanation and an apology if required, even if it is not the organisation/health care professional who is at fault. Always thank the complainant for their time and willingness to let you know about an issue. Make sure that complaints and feedback are dealt with as quickly as possible and taken seriously. All feedback is important, so learn from it at a personal and organisational level.

Minor issues can become major. Major issues may result in more unhappiness and complaints. If complaints are unresolved or mishandled, they can result in litigation.

Finally, it is important to seek help if you are struggling with the emotional impact of facing a complaint. You need to look after your emotional well-being so that you can continue to do your best for your patients.

REFERENCE

1. https://www.legislation.gov.uk/ukpga/2006/29/section/2.

17

Documentation/Record keeping

Without a doubt, we will be judged on the clinical record. Contemporaneous notes are invaluable for determining what occurred with the care of a patient who has run into problems.

Clinical record keeping is an integral component of good professional practice and the delivery of safe health care. It is also a protective shield against criticism of the care provided.

Whatever form records take, whether electronic or paper, good clinical record keeping will facilitate continuity of care and enhance communication within and without the multidisciplinary team.

Remember that patients are entitled to access their records, and any omissions or lacking areas may fuel a potential complaint or even litigation.

As soon as litigation commences, there is an obligation for full and open disclosure. Disclosure obligations are onerous and wide ranging. Emails sent about a patient to a secretary can and will likely be disclosed. Nursing notes that clinicians have never read or seen will form part of the patient's records and the bundle of documents provided to the lawyers and medical experts to dissect and peruse.

Illegible records may be looked upon critically and may be misconstrued as hurried, careless or substandard care.

WHY GOOD RECORD KEEPING IS IMPORTANT

Clinical records are valuable documents to audit the quality of health care services provided. They can be used to audit your own clinical decision making and help with appraisal.

Anyone who has ever done any retrospective research will appreciate the difficulties in collecting and analysing data if the clinical record is incomplete.

Most importantly, in the context of this book, they can be used for investigating serious incidents, patient complaints and litigation cases.

DOI: 10.1201/9781003179351-21

Continuity in clinical notes is of vital importance to patient care, as many different health care professionals are involved in the treatment of a single patient, and they will use the information from other professionals to aid their own decision-making process.

The patient will also benefit through less time lost on repeating tests and by providing information that may prevent inaccurate diagnoses or inappropriate management.

The Caldicott Report, an NHS report on patient information, stated that 'the duty to share information can be as important as the duty to protect patient confidentiality'. Therefore, we need to document the information in a way that can speedily and easily be accessed and understood by fellow health care professionals.

EMERGENCY SITUATIONS

Record keeping in emergency situations can be harder to get right. If a patient's condition is rapidly changing or deteriorating, then the clinical care of the patient clearly takes precedence over documentation. However, once the dust has settled and the acute situation has resolved, the documentation must be completed.

Often, such situations occur in the middle of the night, with a wide variety of health care professionals involved and several discussions taking place simultaneously between clinicians and between clinicians and family members.

In such acute circumstances where the clinical status can be fluid and the patient at risk of harm, the likelihood of scrutiny of these records will be higher.

Usually, there is great variability in the formats of entries into clinical notes among different health care professionals and hospitals, which each have a different patient record system. The various electronic patient records in use across the UK, which cannot speak to each other, seem to make no sense.

The amount and type of information recorded is influenced by the health care professional's seniority, experience, involvement in previous incidents (e.g. if they have been involved in litigation before) and the specific circumstances/setting of the clinical record (i.e. acute admission versus ward round).

Poor documentation can directly lead to allegations of negligence.

FAILURE TO CONSIDER

You can be wrong by dismissing a diagnosis which ultimately proves to be the correct one but you will be worse off if you are seen not to consider the diagnosis in the first place.

Below is an example of a common allegation against health professionals.

Allegation: 'Dr Bloggs failed to consider a diagnosis of deep vein thrombosis (DVT) despite three attendances to the hospital, which represents a breach of duty'.

Indeed, faced with a case where a leg is swollen and red, it would be a breach of duty not to *consider* a DVT within the differential diagnosis. The clinician may argue that they considered a DVT but deemed a cellulitic process to be more likely. However, without documentation, there is no evidence to support that assertion and thought process.

Claimant's lawyer: 'Nowhere is there any documentation regarding the possibility that the claimant may be having a thrombosis of his leg. The assertions by the defendants that a DVT was considered are without any supporting evidence'.

Had the clinician simply written down the differential diagnosis of DVT and then excluded it for reasons that are reasonable, albeit ultimately incorrect, then there would have been a defence.

Defendant's lawyer: 'Dr Bloggs clearly considered the diagnosis of DVT on 3 February but discounted it because the clinical features did not fit with it'.

'REMEMBER, IF YOU DID NOT WRITE IT DOWN, IT DID NOT HAPPEN'

This adage remains reasonably true; however, there is some scope for standard practice to be accepted by the court if there is a weight of evidence behind the assertion.

THE CRITICAL NOTE

Good record keeping is vital at all times, but there are critical times when it is even more vital.

When playing the odds, the likelihood of a complaint or litigation increases dramatically when things do not go to plan or when a diagnosis or management plan is not clear cut or runs some inherent degree of risk.

In these circumstances, a bit of extra attention to the clinical record is vital.

If an operation is complicated, then detailed records are essential to explain to someone assessing the case years later to determine what happened. If nerve damage has occurred, then detailing why and how it occurred may offer significant protection from an allegation of breach of duty.

Compare:

'The inferior hypothetical nerve root was inadvertently partially transected' to

'Adhesions around the lesion were dissected carefully. The medial artery was moved to one side, but scar tissue pulled the inferior hypothetical nerve into the surgical field. This was hidden by a significant venous ooze and was inadvertently damaged during the dissection process'.

Which is more likely to result in criticism from a medical expert, a lay person or a judge?

THE TELEPHONE CALL

The clinical record documents: 'D/W Orthopaedic Registrar. Advises collar and cuff and return to fracture clinic on Monday morning'.

Statement of the emergency medicine doctor: 'I called the registrar and made it clear that the claimant had a fracture dislocation of his shoulder, and even when it was repositioned, there was still some neurological deficit'.

Statement of the orthopaedic registrar: 'I was called by the emergency medicine doctor and told that it was a straightforward dislocated shoulder, which was replaced without complication'.

Such statements are often made years after the index events when neither doctor has much recollection of the events. Who should the court believe?

Records should be ideally kept from both sides of the conversation. These contemporaneous detailed records will protect all parties involved and provide valuable information for any root cause analysis. Each side should record what information was provided and what clinical decision was made.

Patient phone calls should be documented effectively, with names, dates, content and actions taken in response to the patient's call. It is also important to make notes regarding out-of-hours phone calls and any consultations with colleagues about the patient's case. These should be transcribed or incorporated into the patient's notes as soon as possible.

PRACTICALITIES OF RECORD KEEPING

Every entry in the medical record should be dated, timed and legible.

Each should be signed by the person making the entry, with a clear name and position. Records should be made as soon as possible after the event to be documented.

If there is a delay, the time of the event and the delay should be recorded as well as the reasons for the delay.

Abbreviations may cause confusion if they are not standard, or they may be confused with other conditions.

Clinical records should be objective and focused on the relevant clinical findings and decisions.

Historically, terms such as stating the patient's condition was 'supratentorial' cropped up in the medical record to suggest the condition was psychological or fabricated. Any flippant comments or remarks will be questioned, and what may appear humorous when written will not be when explained to a judge assessing a clinical negligence case.

For correction of any errors, draw a single line through the entry, document the correct info, add the date and time and sign off on the correction.

Never ever alter the clinical record. It is not worth it and can result in referral to the GMC.

Labelling a patient can result in a complaint, so be cautious about labelling someone as a malingerer or an alcoholic without definitive evidence to support such assertions.

LEGAL AND REGULATORY ISSUES

The Good Medical Practice guidelines issued by the GMC clearly state that clinical records represent a formal record of the clinician's work and must be clear, accurate, legible and written in a scientific manner.

They should include all relevant clinical findings and a record of the decisions made and actions agreed, as well as the identity of the clinician who made the decisions and agreed to the actions, a record of the information given to the patient and a record of any drugs prescribed and other investigations or treatments performed.

Confidentiality and data protection are becoming more important, and breaches carry significant penalties. Clinical records, including any patient identifiable information and data on the diagnosis, prognosis or treatment of any patient or subject, are considered confidential and personal data. These data can only be shared with the prior written consent of the data subject to the data manager.

In certain circumstances, confidentiality can be breached in the public interest if failure to disclose such information may expose others to a risk of death or serious harm, such as reporting gunshot wounds, acts of terrorism, risks of serious communicable disease transmission and concerns relating to the ability to drive a motor vehicle.

THE GENERAL DATA PROTECTION REGULATION

The GDPR requires the implementation of effective controls across the six privacy principles of:

- Lawfulness, fairness and transparency
- Purpose limitation
- Data minimisation
- Accuracy
- Storage limitation
- Integrity and confidentiality

The GDPR is designed to ensure that individuals have more control over their personal data and gives them the following rights:

- To be informed about how their personal data are processed
- Access to their personal data and details of how they are processed
- Rectification of inaccuracies in a timely manner
- Erasure of their personal data ('right to be forgotten')
- To restrict processing of their personal data
- To obtain their personal data and reuse them for their own purposes ('data portability')
- To object to the processing of their personal data
- Not to be subject to automated decision making and profiling

Medical practice is highly impacted, as we process, document and communicate a large volume of sensitive personal data, which are used for the purposes of patient care, health management and scientific research.

All health care staff, trusts and private hospitals in the UK must undergo mandatory training in this element of data protection, as it is an important part of appraisal.

JOHNSTONE V NHS GRAMPIAN: DOCUMENTARY EVIDENCE OUTWEIGHS ORAL EVIDENCE IN CONSENT CASE

A patient underwent transsphenoidal surgery in Aberdeen Royal Infirmary in January 2011 to treat a pituitary tumour believed to be responsible for excreting excessive levels of growth hormone. Prior to this, it had been treated conservatively without any major issues.

The procedure was complicated by post-operative cerebral spinal fluid (CSF) leakage and meningitis. A further procedure was required, and the patient had to take medication for the rest of his life.

The patient alleged that the surgeons he met in the lead-up to the surgery failed in their duty of care to him by failing to explain the material risks involved in the surgery. They also allegedly failed to provide more information on the alternative options of treatment by way of radiosurgery or continuing conservative treatment and the risks attached to these. The surgical team disagreed and argued that this information had been provided.

The judge considered that each side's witnesses could not be said to be more reliable and/or credible over the other, so it was necessary to decide the case by drawing inferences from the documentary evidence presented during the trial. The judge found a note, dictated by one of the surgeons soon after the meeting with the patient, to be a fair and accurate summary of the discussions.

It detailed the options of surgery and radiosurgery, their respective pros and cons and the risks of surgery, including the risk of post-operative CSF leakage, meningitis and future surgery.

The patient denied this discussion had happened, but this assertion was rejected based on the contemporaneous note.

This emphasises the importance of documentation, and in this case, the whole judgement depended upon it. The judge found both testimonies convincing and could not decide whose recollections were more accurate. The judge could have made a positive judgement based on the clinical notes but could also have made a detrimental judgement if information was conspicuously absent.

As well as highlighting the need for accurate and comprehensive notes, this case also points out that whoever 'acts' more convincingly on the day will be more likely to be believed. The truth is key, and the court will likely see through attempts at deception, which can be damaging. Conduct in court will be considered in another section.

The old adage of 'if it's not written in the notes, it didn't happen' is true to some degree. Clinician testimony is still considered, but it is an uphill struggle to convince the court that something happened when it is not documented. This is compounded by the testimony of poor patients who, regardless of whether there was a breach of duty or not, have come to harm.

However, if you are documenting a discussion or an action, then it is vital that this actually occurred. A potentially greater injustice is clinical documentation which seems to prove conversations surrounding, for example, consent, which never happened. This is not only unjust but serious professional misconduct. Honesty is a vital pillar of all health care professionals.

18

Professional obligations and the role of reflections

When you are in the business of saving lives, hurting anybody, even unintentionally, can leave a mark. Self-criticism and self-reflection are great tools to correct ourselves. Hence, it is crucial for doctors to be able to reflect on the treatments they provide, the decisions they make and the actions they take in their professional capacity. The appraisal and revalidation process helps facilitate this process.

While reflecting and considering how you could have prevented an error may be helpful in preventing future errors, going through unnecessary stress over what has already happened can be destructive. Self-reflection in a rational manner is challenging when life and death situations are involved. At times, it may be difficult to separate one's personal feelings from a professional situation. It is especially hard to avoid professional guilt.

It is important not only to reflect on which events went well or badly but also on how you felt at the time and how this experience has impacted how you practise medicine. In medicine, there is always more to learn, more mistakes to be made and more progress to be made.

Although self-reflection is currently stated not to be accepted as proof in court, there is no guarantee. Moreover, when a physician is defending themselves in court, self-reflection may seem similar to admission of guilt. To put it simply, the physician should also have a sense of self-preservation in addition to the duty of candour.

The Bawa-Garba case sent shockwaves through the medical world when her personal reflections were used against her as evidence of recognition of poor clinical care. The GMC have subsequently sought to assure the medical profession that they will not use personal reflections in fitness to practise proceedings. However, when legal proceedings ensue, all relevant materials are disclosable, and this may include personal reflections if within a formal record.

DOI: 10.1201/9781003179351-22

SECTION 5

Dealing with litigation

19

Medical defence organisations

The GMC Good Medical Practice (GMP) guidance, Section 63, requires that health care professionals in the UK have appropriate insurance or indemnity arrangements covering the full scope of their medical practice.

> You must make sure you have adequate insurance or indemnity cover so that your patients will not be disadvantaged if they make a claim about the clinical care you have provided in the UK.
>
> *(Domain 4: Maintaining Trust – Ethical Guidance – GMC)*

Many choose to join an MDO for this purpose.

MDOs are unregulated, independent, membership-based organisations. They are typically funded by membership fees.

MDOs provide medical professionals with access to advice, assistance and representation in a range of legal and ethical matters.

THE ROLE OF A MEDICAL DEFENCE ORGANISATION

The main role of an MDO is to protect its members from litigation, professional misconduct investigations and other legal challenges that may arise during the course of their practice.

MDOs typically offer a range of services to their members to help them manage the risks and challenges associated with medical practice and to ensure they provide the best possible care to their patients. Such services include:

- *Legal advice and representation*: An MDO provides legal advice and representation to its members in the event of a claim or complaint. This can include assistance with preparing a defence, negotiating a settlement and representation in court.

- *Indemnity cover*: An MDO provides its members with indemnity cover, which means that the MDO may cover the cost of any compensation

DOI: 10.1201/9781003179351-24

awarded against the member as a result of a claim or complaint up to a certain limit.

- *Complaints and investigations*: An MDO can provide support and guidance to its members if they are the subject of a complaint or investigation. This can include assistance with responding to the complaint, preparing for an investigation and representation at hearings or meetings.

- *Training and education*: An MDO can provide its members with access to training and education on various topics related to medical practice. This can include training on clinical risk management, ethical issues and legal requirements.

- *Advice on regulatory and professional issues*: An MDO can provide advice and guidance to its members on regulatory and professional issues, such as compliance with professional standards, disciplinary proceedings and fitness to practise.

In addition to supporting individual health care professionals, MDOs may also advocate for changes to health care policies and regulations that impact the medical profession as a whole. This can include lobbying for reforms to improve patient safety, reduce regulatory burdens and ensure fair and equitable treatment of health care professionals.

ACCESSING SUPPORT FROM A MEDICAL DEFENCE ORGANISATION

Many MDOs provide a helpline that members can call for advice and support on a range of issues, such as legal or ethical questions, complaints or investigations and other professional issues. Members also have access to numerous online resources, such as guidance documents, case studies and training materials, which can be accessed either through the MDO's website or a member portal.

MDOs may organise meetings, seminars and other events where members can network with other health care professionals, learn about the latest developments in their field and receive training and education.

If a member is faced with a claim or complaint, they can contact their MDO for support and guidance. The MDO typically assigns a case handler or solicitor to manage a member's case. The case handler provides advice on how to respond to the claim or complaint and may provide legal representation if necessary.

A WARNING ABOUT INDEMNITY COVER

The indemnity provided by an MDO is a form of insurance that protects medical professionals, such as doctors, dentists and other health care practitioners, against medical negligence claims.

If a member faces a claim, the MDO may provide financial support to cover the cost of any compensation awarded against the member, as well as any legal fees or other costs associated with the claim.

The level of indemnity cover provided by an MDO varies, depending on the type of membership, the individual circumstances of the member and their area of practice. Some MDOs provide a set level of cover for all members, while others offer a range of options for members to choose from.

However, the indemnity cover provided by an MDO is usually discretionary, meaning that *the MDO is not obligated to provide cover in all circumstances.* For example, an MDO may decline cover for claims arising from deliberate or criminal acts. As long as the decision to decline indemnity is not malicious or irrational, there is no appeal against that exercise of discretion, and it is not possible to enforce a right to indemnity.

While medical professionals working in the NHS are covered by crown indemnity,[1] those working outside the NHS, with some limited exceptions, are not and thus require indemnity cover. The discretionary nature of indemnity cover provided by MDOs can be problematic, as members of MDOs may find themselves without the necessary financial support in the event of a claim or complaint being made against them, and patients may be left without the ability to seek compensation for any harm suffered.

In 2018, the Medical Defence Union (MDU) exercised its discretion and declined to indemnify rogue surgeon Ian Paterson, prompting the government to launch a consultation on indemnity cover for regulated health care professionals. The consultation aimed to determine whether legislation was necessary to require all medical professionals who are not covered by crown indemnity to hold regulated insurance-like indemnity rather than relying on the unregulated discretionary indemnity provided by the MDOs.

The government was concerned that, unlike commercial insurance companies, MDOs have no contractual obligation to meet the cost of any claim against the members they cover and no legal obligation to ensure that they have the reserves to cover the cost of claims, raising the risk that patients will be unable to access appropriate compensation. Furthermore, MDOs are not obligated to disclose their complete financial status, which can leave health care professionals unaware of the risk of their discretionary indemnity provider refusing to provide cover due to inadequate finances.

MDOs are also not subject to regulation on financial conduct and fair treatment by the Financial Conduct Authority and Prudential Regulation Authority, potentially leaving members at risk of unfair treatment. The responses to the consultation were published in December 2022,[2] and the government has said that it will continue to work closely with stakeholders on these issues.

CHOOSING A MEDICAL DEFENCE ORGANISATION

There are several MDOs in the UK, and the main ones include:

- *MDU*: This is one of the largest MDOs in the UK, offering membership to doctors, dentists and other health care professionals. A not-for-profit organisation, it has been operating for more than 130 years.

- *Medical Protection Society (MPS)*: This is another large MDO. Established in 1892, the MPS has members not just in the UK but worldwide.

- *Medical and Dental Defence Union of Scotland (MDDUS)*: This MDO, set up in 1902, offers membership to health care professionals in Scotland and across the UK. The MDDUS was established as a private company but is operated as a mutual membership organisation.

While the services offered by MDOs are broadly similar, each MDO has its unique approach. Health care professionals should carefully consider their options when choosing an MDO. Factors to consider may include the cost of membership, level of indemnity cover provided, quality of legal and medicolegal advice and availability of training and education.

NOTES

1. In England, this is through their trust's membership in the CNST administered by the NHS Resolution. In Wales, indemnity is provided through the CNST and Health Board by Welsh Risk Pool Services. In Scotland, indemnity is provided by the Clinical Negligence and Other Risks Indemnity Scheme. In Northern Ireland, each health and social care trust provides its own indemnity, funded by the Department of Health, Social Security and Public Safety.
2. https://www.gov.uk/government/consultations/appropriate-clinical-negligence-cover/public-feedback/appropriate-clinical-negligence-cover-summary-of-responses.

20

Captain of the ship

Who should take the blame when a patient comes to harm? Clearly, the answer is highly dependent upon the circumstances of the harm and the background therein.

Should a senior – for example, a consultant – accept responsibility for the whole team under them? If a junior on the consultant's team makes an error, should the consultant be accountable for it? If a junior calls the consultant for advice and the patient comes to harm despite that advice or even because of it, who should take the blame?

When considering care under the NHS, the question is not so vital, as crown indemnity tends to apply, and the trust as a whole is held responsible. This does not protect individuals completely, and clinicians are vulnerable to disciplinary action or even allegations of negligent manslaughter in the worst scenarios. However, the team is held liable in most cases.

The private sector is slightly different, as junior doctors are not usually involved. The team is larger, and often, Resident Medical Officers (RMOs) are involved in care for private patients.

Clinical errors are easier to pinpoint and lay blame for. Non-clinical errors are harder to define. For example, non-technical errors in the operating theatre can cause disputes between parties over where the blame/fault lies. In the theatre, surgeons are part of a multidisciplinary team who all work to ensure that the patient remains safe. Things do go wrong, and they go wrong for a myriad of reasons; for example, moving and handling incidents, retained instruments or swabs and intraoperative injuries to the patient, such as diathermy burns.

If the scrub practitioner hands the surgeon a faulty piece of equipment and they use it, and the patient comes to harm, who is responsible? The surgeon or the scrub practitioner? Indeed, if the scrub practitioner was in turn handed the faulty equipment by a circulating nurse, where does the blame lie?

THE HISTORY OF CAPTAIN OF THE SHIP

Captain of the ship was first introduced into the law of negligence by a case in the United States, McConnell v Williams, 361 Pa. 355 (1949). An obstetrician

DOI: 10.1201/9781003179351-25

asked an intern 'to be his assistant and take care of the baby at the time of the delivery'. The delivery was difficult and required the obstetrician's complete attention. When the child was delivered, the obstetrician turned the child over to the intern for the purpose of tying the cord and applying a solution of silver nitrate into the infant's eyes. Applying silver nitrate was a regularly established practice in obstetrical cases and was required by the rules and regulations of the Department of Health of the Commonwealth of Pennsylvania.

One of the nurses present in the operating room noticed that the intern filled the syringe and squirted the solution once into the child's left eye and twice into the right eye, putting too much of the solution into the right eye and failing to irrigate, which resulted in lost sight.

The only question in the case was whether the surgeon should be responsible for the negligence of the intern, i.e. the surgeon was the captain of the ship and had overall responsibility. At the trial, the court listened to all the evidence and then dismissed the case against the surgeon.

The Scottish Court of Session judgement in Andrews v Greater Glasgow Health Board [2019] CSOH 31 addressed the scope of the duty of care of a junior doctor. This case concerned the death of an elderly lady caused by an ischaemic bowel. She had attended hospital by ambulance with symptoms of chest and upper epigastric pain, vomiting and diarrhoea. The investigations were mostly normal, and she was discharged by the junior doctor with a diagnosis of viral gastroenteritis. Prior to her discharge, the junior doctor discussed the deceased's case with the on-call consultant, who approved the decision. Her symptoms developed, and following a return to hospital, ischaemic bowel secondary to superior mesenteric artery thrombosis was noted. A laparotomy confirmed significant necrosis, and resection was unfortunately not possible.

With regard to negligence, it was found that it should have been recognised that the deceased might be suffering from a serious medical condition and that the junior doctor failed to advise her that she should be admitted to hospital and breached his duty of care.

Furthermore, it was found that the junior doctor had provided the consultant with inaccurate information about the deceased and her circumstances, which he had to be held responsible for.

The defence tried to rely on a passage in Jones' Medical Negligence (5th edition, paragraph 3.115), which stated that 'inexperienced doctors will discharge their duties of care by seeking the assistance of their superiors to check their work, even though they may themselves have made a mistake'.

This argument was rejected, and the finding was that 'in general, the principle is that a junior and inexperienced doctor must achieve the same standard of care as a more experienced colleague would be expected to bring to the task in hand'.

The judge in this case also considered the English decision of FB v Rana [2017] in which the Court of Appeal held that in taking a case history, a junior doctor did not hold a lesser duty than a more experienced colleague. The Court of Appeal held that a doctor is to be judged by the standard of skill and care appropriate to the post that they are fulfilling and not their experience.

Captaincy rests on the surgeon's ability to exercise practical control over the work being done by a hospital employee in a way that is significant enough to bring them under their professional umbrella. Could and should the surgeon have done something to prevent the harm? Clearly, the surgeon is reliant on ancillary staff, but acting recklessly and not engaging with the staff or ensuring that they have fulfilled their mandatory safety obligations can be criticised. The duty of the doctor is to do everything in their power to protect the patient, and failure to do so can be an avenue for litigation.

SO WHO IS RESPONSIBLE?

Patient safety is the overriding principle of the duty of care we have as medical professionals. We all need to work towards keeping our patients safe and doing no harm.

In the operating theatre, the surgeon arguably has ultimate responsibility for their patients during the procedure. However, anaesthetists may be considered responsible for issues with the anaesthetic, airway or equipment relating to the provision of anaesthesia. Anaesthetists also hold a level of responsibility for moving and handling, as well as aspects of care where changes in the patient should be alerted to the surgeon; for example, a dropping blood pressure that may indicate a bleed.

While the theatre staff should usually be responsible for ensuring that the correct equipment for the operation is available, the surgeon should be satisfied that this has been done correctly, particularly if there are specific technical or product requirements. There should also be provision of equipment for potential complications. All of these requirements should be checked at the pre-surgery brief, which should be led by the consultant surgeon.

The World Health Organization (WHO) checklist defines equipment issues or concerns under the responsibility of the nursing team. However, it is the surgeon's responsibility to try and minimise the risk of harm. Failure to engage with the staff and check with them regarding the equipment that will or may be required may be criticised. If the surgeon could have done something to avoid harm but did not, then that may be seen as a breach of duty.

If an operating surgeon has the ability to give orders to influence staff conduct or to get more information from the staff, and that conduct or information is needed for safe patient care, then it is reasonable to expect that the doctor will make those requests and fair to hold them liable if they do not do so. A patient can rightly expect them to take all reasonable steps to keep them safe if it is within their ability to do so.

Another grey area regarding the attribution of blame is medication administration, such as the administration of antibiotics or provision of thromboprophylaxis. If a drug is written up for pre-operative administration and the nursing teams fail to administer, can the operating surgeon be completely absolved of responsibility, or should they have checked that it had been given prior to commencing surgery?

Delegable versus non-delegable duties

Some duties can be reasonably delegated to other professionals, such as the administration of prescribed medication. Other duties are non-delegable, such as ensuring that no swabs are left in the surgical wound. Granted, the surgeon is reliant on the assistance of the nursing staff to undertake counts; however, the overall responsibility is the surgeon's. The patient is asleep and reliant on the surgeon for their safety.

The General Medical Council's view

The GMP by the GMC states that doctors must take prompt action if they think that patient safety, dignity or comfort is or may be seriously compromised. If patients are at risk because of inadequate premises, equipment or other resources, policies or systems, the matter should be put right if possible. Concerns must be raised in line with the guidance and the workplace's policy. The steps taken should also be recorded.

Often, statements from staff members highlight failings in the system, but these should be raised before harm occurs. Ultimately, a clinician may be criticised for not raising concerns and yet proceeding to practise in an unsafe environment, thereby putting their patients in the way of foreseeable harm.

WORLD HEALTH ORGANIZATION CHECKLIST

The Royal College of Surgeons guidance, Good Surgical Practice, identifies that in order to ensure consistency in patient safety, the surgeon should be fully compliant with the principles and practice of the WHO Surgical Safety Checklist (2008) and its adaptation through the Five Steps to Safer Surgery (National Patient Safety Agency, 2010). Failure to undertake such tasks can be considered a breach of duty, as they are part of the standard of care expected.

Below are some examples of such failures

Retained swabs and foreign material left behind sadly still occurs. Surgical pathways should ensure that swabs and instruments are counted, and this responsibility is held by the nursing staff. However, it is ultimately the surgeon's responsibility to ensure that the count has been done.

They cannot be held accountable for an inaccurate count but can be held accountable for not asking for or facilitating the count or ignoring a concern regarding the count, as this would be substandard practice.

A CASE IN POINT: Loose Cannula

In one case, a scrub practitioner handed an ophthalmic surgeon a cannula on a 2 mL Luer lock syringe. The cannula was introduced into the eye, and the injection commenced. The cannula flew off the syringe and caused significant damage to the eye, resulting in poor vision. The cannula was not adequately secured by the scrub nurse. Then, it was not appropriately tightened by the scrub practitioner, and it was not tested by the operating surgeon. The blame clearly lay with both; however, it was not the scrub practitioner who placed the cannula in the eye but the surgeon. The whole incident and the harm could have been avoided by the operating surgeon checking the tightness of the cannula before subjecting the patient to the risk of foreseeable harm.

A CASE IN POINT: Diathermy Burn

Another example is the potential for a diathermy burn. Incorrectly connecting a diathermy or resting it on the patient and thus causing inadvertent burns can result in harm. It is not the surgeon's responsibility to connect the equipment, but failing to recognise an issue and working with the staff to determine a problem and prevent harm may be a criticism raised against surgeons.

The undeniable overarching aim of a doctor is to care for the patient and do everything within their reasonable control to minimise the risk of harm. The doctor relies on the staff around them to assist, and it is inevitable that they will delegate some of the care to those individuals. A doctor needs to be confident in the processes being followed and the ability of those staff. They need to make sure that any weaknesses are addressed and cooperate and assist the staff in doing their job and protecting the patient.

If the court finds that the clinician could have done things differently and avoided harm, then they may be criticised. The captain of the ship doctrine does not apply to UK law, but some of the principles can be carried over.

A patient is usually under the ultimate care of a consultant, and that consultant/senior doctor owes them a mostly non-delegable duty of care. It has to be honoured, and if a doctor fails to undertake steps that were within their reasonable power to uphold this duty to keep their patient safe, then they may be criticised or held liable.

21

What is disclosure, and what is disclosable in a medical negligence case?

During court proceedings, disclosure refers to the process of sharing relevant documents and information with other parties involved in the case. This includes providing all documents relevant to the case to ensure fairness and transparency in the legal process.

The disclosure process is governed by court rules and procedures, and failure to comply with these and to disclose relevant information can result in penalties and adverse judgements.

The test for the scope of disclosure is not relevance but necessity, i.e. whether disclosure is necessary for fairly deciding the proceedings.[1]

WHAT IS DISCLOSURE?

A party discloses a document by stating that the document exists or has existed.[2] 'Document' means anything in which information of any description is recorded[3] and therefore includes photographs, videos, audio, meta-data and physical objects.

Standard disclosure requires that a party discloses all documents on which they rely and all documents that adversely affect their own case, adversely affect another party's case or support another party's case, unless such documents are protected by the principles of legal privilege.

To provide disclosure, the disclosing party must make a reasonable search for such documents. The duty of disclosure is limited to documents that are or have been in the party's control.[4]

DOI: 10.1201/9781003179351-26

Examples of documents that form part of the defendant's disclosure in medical negligence claims are:

- Medical records, including clinical notes; nursing notes; operation notes and consent forms; laboratory reports, request forms and results; radiology images and reports; photographs, audio and visual records' documentation; correspondence, such as emails; and all other personal data held by the health care providers
- Patient leaflets
- Relevant protocols and guidelines
- The complaint file (if any), which includes all draft documents, email correspondence and witness evidence
- SUI reports and any documentation emanating therefrom, including minutes of interviews, witness evidence and earlier drafts
- The clinician's e-portfolio and reflections entries
- The clinician's curriculum vitae and training records

The court may make an order for specific disclosure.[5] Such an order may be made before proceedings have begun, though that would be unusual.

Once proceedings have begun, the duty of disclosure continues until the case is concluded.[6]

DISCLOSURE STATEMENT

Usually, disclosure is given by way of a standard court document called a List of Documents (Form N265). This is usually drafted by the legal team.

INSPECTION OF DOCUMENTS

Once a party states that a particular document exists or has existed, the other party has the right to inspect that document, unless the document is no longer in the control of the party who discloses it,[7] unless it is disproportionate to the issues in the case to permit inspection[8] or unless there is a right to withhold inspection.[9]

Documents may be withheld on the grounds that disclosure would damage the public interest.[10]

Documents may also be withheld on the grounds of legal privilege. Legal privilege refers to the principle that certain documents or communications are protected from disclosure to the other party in legal proceedings. This applies to confidential communications between a lawyer and their client or a third party (e.g. expert) for the primary purpose of preparing or conducting litigation. This privilege covers documents and communications that are created or obtained for the purposes of litigation or in anticipation of litigation.

Legal privilege is not an absolute right. There are exceptions, such as if the client consents to disclosure or if there is an overriding public interest in disclosure.

During court proceedings, a party may, at various stages, choose to waive legal privilege and serve, for example, factual statements from witnesses who have relevant information about the case and expert reports prepared by independent experts who have been instructed to provide their opinion on the case, notwithstanding that such documents have been prepared for the specific purpose of litigation.

USE OF DISCLOSURE

Documents disclosed are confidential unless and until referred to at a court hearing held in public, the court gives permission or it is agreed otherwise.

THE IMPORTANCE OF CONTEMPORANEOUS RECORDS

The GMC emphasises the importance of keeping contemporaneous, accurate and comprehensive medical records. According to the GMC's GMP guidance, doctors must keep clear and accurate patient records, including all relevant clinical findings, decisions made, information given to patients and any drugs or treatment given. The guidance also highlights that doctors should make records at the time events occurred or as soon as possible afterwards. They should ensure their records are up to date, reflect the patient's condition accurately and are accessible to others who are providing care or treatment to the patient.

The GMC further emphasises that keeping good medical records is not only a professional responsibility but also a legal requirement and that doctors must make sure their records accurately reflect the care they provided. The GMC warns that failure to keep adequate medical records may result in complaints and investigations, as well as allegations of inadequate professional performance or serious professional misconduct.

MDOs also recognise the importance of good medical record keeping. For example, the MDU advises its members that keeping accurate and up-to-date medical records is essential for good clinical care, as well as for legal, regulatory and professional reasons. The MDU guidance emphasises the importance of recording clinical findings, diagnoses, treatments and outcomes in addition to any discussions with patients, decisions made and risks involved. Records should be legible, dated and signed. Any alterations or additions should be clearly marked and explained.

Health care professionals may have to rely on what they have recorded in medical records, in numerous scenarios; for example, clinical audits, complaints, statements for the coroner, disciplinary proceedings and reports to manage medical negligence claims.

Medical records are considered a crucial piece of evidence in medical negligence cases and are often seen as an objective and reliable source of information. Therefore, it is essential for health care professionals to maintain accurate and complete medical records. If information is missing or inaccurate, claims that could have been defended may have to be settled.

Before making a final decision, the court considers all evidence. This includes medical records, factual witness testimonies and expert witness evidence. When assessing the credibility of a health care professional's testimony, the court may also consider the quality of the medical records and attach substantial importance to them. These records can, therefore, play a significant role in shaping the court's decision in a case.

Health care professionals are advised to follow the following principles when keeping medical records:

- Make detailed contemporaneous records.

- Write the record in the expectation that someone else (e.g. another health care professional, the patient, a lawyer and a coroner/judge) may read it.

- Record all relevant information, including:

  ✓ The patient's previous medical and social history
  ✓ The patient's presenting symptoms
  ✓ All examinations undertaken and their findings
  ✓ All investigations ordered and their results
  ✓ The differential diagnoses
  ✓ The working diagnosis
  ✓ Discussions with the patient about their condition, treatment options, risks and benefits, and any other relevant information
  ✓ Any discussions with colleagues
  ✓ The treatment plan
  ✓ Consent for treatments and procedures
  ✓ The plan for follow-up care

- Sign and date all records, whether handwritten or electronic.

- Ensure that the information can be easily understood by other health care professionals by using clear and concise language and writing legibly. All records should be objective and free from personal opinions or biases.

- Keep records up to date and ensure that medical records are regularly updated with new information, including changes in the patient's condition or the treatment plan.

- Beware of electronic records that automatically populate and tick boxes. These are no substitute for proper record keeping.

- If corrections need to be made to a medical record, clearly mark these as such and document the reason for the correction.

As accurate and clear medical records are crucial for any medicolegal defence, it is important for health care professionals to incorporate these tips into their daily practice.

NOTES

1. Science Research Council v Nasse [1980] AC 1028.
2. CPR 31.2.
3. CPR 31.4.
4. CPR 31.8.
5. CPR 31.12.
6. CPR 31.11.
7. CPR 31.3(1)(a).
8. CPR 31.3(2).
9. CPR 31.3(1)(b).
10. CPR 31.19(1).

22

The legal process and the relationship with your lawyer

Health care professionals may occasionally find themselves involved in legal matters, including medical negligence claims. While this can be an intimidating experience, it is important to remember that a compensation claim is not about assigning blame. Most health care professionals will encounter a compensation claim at some stage in their career.

When faced with such situations, the health care professional must understand the process and the dynamics of their relationship with their legal team. By doing so, they can navigate the legal proceedings more effectively and alleviate some of the associated anxieties.

THE INTIMATION OF A CLAIM

A health care professional may become aware of a potential claim in a number of ways, such as:

- There may have been an internal investigation (e.g. complaint review or incident investigation) that identified failings in the care provided and the possibility of a claim.

- The patient or their family may directly inform the health care professional about their intention to bring a claim. This may be in a conversation where they express dissatisfaction with the treatment received or through formal written correspondence.

- The patient's legal representatives may correspond with the health care professional directly. This is more common in relation to care provided by GPs and private treatment.

- The patient or their legal representative may request copies of their medical records and any other associated records or documents.

DOI: 10.1201/9781003179351-27

- The trust or hospital may advise the health care professional of a claim notified. This may be through formal channels, such as the legal or risk management department.

If the health care professional becomes aware of a potential claim, it is vital that this is reported through the appropriate channels.

NHS settings should have clear policies and protocols for how to report a potential claim. If in doubt, start with the trust's legal department, and they will be able to advise further. The NHS Resolution's reporting guidelines[1] set out when a trust should notify a claim to them and how. Notification is undertaken by the trust's in-house legal team, who may need input from the health care professionals involved in the case.

The NHS Resolution expects the trust to preserve relevant notes, records and other key documentation; to respond promptly to requests for instructions; and to keep those involved updated as to the progress of a particular claim and its outcome. Once notified, the NHS Resolution decides whether to handle matters in house or to appoint panel solicitors on a full or limited basis.

In a **private setting**, advice should be sought from the Medical Defence Organisation (MDO) immediately, and the MDO will advise on the next steps. The MDO team managing the case usually includes a doctor, a case handler and sometimes a solicitor. They will want to see notes and any other documents that may be relevant. These should be provided promptly. Usually, the MDO will write to the claimant's solicitors to confirm their representation and will ask the claimant's solicitors not to communicate directly with the health care professional but to correspond via the MDO.

THE INITIAL INTERACTION WITH THE LEGAL TEAM AND THE IMPORTANCE OF HONESTY

During the initial interaction with their legal team, health care professionals should feel comfortable disclosing all relevant facts. Lawyers are bound by professional ethics and legal obligations to maintain the confidentiality of information shared. By upholding client privilege, lawyers provide a secure and protected space for health care professionals to share sensitive details without fear of adverse consequences. This privilege extends to any initial witness statements provided, as well as any legal advice received. This means that such communications cannot be disclosed to third parties without the consent of the health care professional.

It is crucial that health care professionals engage openly and honestly with their legal team so that the legal team can assess the situation, evaluate the potential legal implications and provide appropriate guidance. Any information provided must be accurate and truthful, even if it may be unfavourable or potentially damaging to the case. Withholding or misrepresenting crucial information can significantly compromise the lawyer's ability to advise effectively. Moreover, being forthcoming with all relevant information allows the legal team to address potential challenges and anticipate counterarguments from the opposing party.

Clear and concise communication helps to eliminate misunderstandings and ensures that the legal team is well informed and can give effective advice.

Sharing information promptly is also vital, as it allows the legal team to gather all necessary details and initiate appropriate actions in a timely manner. By providing all relevant details and responding to requests for information in a timely and accurate manner, health care professionals contribute to a strong working relationship with their legal team.

DISCLOSURE

To assess the validity of their case, the patient's solicitors must review all relevant records and information. The majority of these records will be obtained from the health care provider (in an NHS setting) or health care professional (in a private setting). When a disclosure request is made, full disclosure should be given, even if this involves disclosing documents that may be unhelpful to the case.

Providing records and information in a timely and comprehensive manner ensures that the patient's solicitors have access to the necessary documentation to evaluate the claim effectively. The health care professional's cooperation in fulfilling a disclosure request plays a crucial role in enabling a fair and thorough assessment of the case.

THE LETTER OF CLAIM

If, after the disclosure of records and taking expert advice, the claimant decides to proceed with a claim, their solicitors will send a letter of claim. This serves as the formal initiation of the legal process. It is typically prepared by the claimant's lawyer and is addressed to the defendant. The letter should be based on independent expert evidence and should contain the following information:

- The claimant's details
- The factual background, including what treatment the claimant received, when and where the claimant received that treatment and who gave that treatment
- The details of the alleged negligence and the resulting injuries and harm

The letter should be comprehensive and factual and clearly articulate the allegations.

The claimant should not issue formal proceedings until 4 months from the date of the letter. This gives the defendant's legal team the opportunity to consider the claim fully.

THE LETTER OF RESPONSE

The defendant must acknowledge receipt of a letter of claim within 14 days and provide a letter of response within 4 months.

Upon receiving the letter of claim, the defendant's legal team should investigate the case and prepare a letter of response. This response provides an opportunity for the defendant to address the allegations and present their position. The defendant should only provide a letter of response supported by independent expert evidence.

The legal team should collaborate with the health care professional and medical experts to gather evidence, assess the merits of the claim and develop a well-reasoned and evidence-based response. If the legal team proposes to make admissions in the letter of response, it is usual practice to seek agreement from the health care professional.

In some cases, the letter of response may admit the claim either in part or in its entirety. In such circumstances, it is usual to then enter settlement negotiations. This allows both parties to explore the possibility of resolving the dispute amicably, potentially avoiding the need for formal court proceedings.

If the claim is denied, the letter of response must provide clear and detailed reasons. This allows the claimant to consider their position and evaluate the strength of their case.

The aim is to ensure that both parties are provided with sufficient information to make informed decisions and have every opportunity to resolve the dispute informally.

Either side can suggest alternative ways of resolving the dispute (e.g. negotiation, mediation or settlement meetings) at any time up to the start of formal proceedings.

COURT PROCEEDINGS

If the dispute remains unresolved following the letter of response, the claimant has the option to initiate legal proceedings, which involve submitting a formal court document known as a claim form. Once the claim form is officially lodged with the court, the claimant has 4 months to serve it upon the defendant. Typically, this is done by post or email to the defendant's legal representatives.

The particulars of claim is a formal document that outlines the precise facts on which the claimant relies and the allegations made against the defendant. In most cases, this is similar to the letter of claim already served.

The defendant's legal team must formally acknowledge receipt of the particulars of claim to the court within 14 days. Failure to do so may result in the court entering judgement against the defendant.

DEFENCE

The defence should be served within 28 days of the proceedings being served, unless an extension is agreed with the claimant. Failure to serve the defence within the required timeframe can result in a court judgement being entered against the defendant.

The defence is the official response to the particulars of claim. It addresses each paragraph and indicates whether it is admitted or denied. If it is denied, a detailed response should be provided.

The defence contains a statement of truth, which verifies its contents. This is usually signed by the trust's legal team or by the legal representative on behalf of the trust. If care was provided privately, the health care professional will be asked to sign the statement of truth. If the document contains a false statement, it may lead to contempt of court.[?] Being in contempt of court is punishable with a fine or maximum penalty of 2 years in prison.

WITNESS STATEMENTS

As the claim progresses, the court will order that factual witness statements be exchanged by the parties.

The defendant will need to serve statements of fact that support their defence. This will include statements from those directly involved in the care of the claimant.

The lawyers draft the witness statements based on interviews and notes with the health care professionals involved. As with the defence, a witness statement requires verification through a statement of truth, which the health care professional will need to sign.

EXPERT REPORTS

Experts are doctors with broad experience in a particular field of medicine and medicolegal work. They are usually still in practice or have recently retired.

Expert reports play a pivotal role in medical negligence cases by providing an objective opinion on the standard of care and, if the care was substandard, whether the substandard care caused harm.

An expert's duty is to advise the court, not the party who instructs them.

Experts give their advice in a written report. The initial report is advisory only and is legally privileged. However, if the case is litigated, the court will order the parties to exchange written reports from their respective nominated experts. Both sides may put written questions to an expert to clarify the report, and the expert must answer these. After time, there will usually be a meeting of experts, and the experts will produce a joint statement stating their respective opinions on the key issues in their expertise. This is a key stage in the case, as it enables the parties to narrow down the issues that are in dispute. Should the case proceed to trial, the expert will give oral evidence at the trial on the issues remaining in dispute.

TRIAL

Only a small number of claims ultimately proceed to trial. If a case does proceed to trial, the factual witnesses will provide evidence, as will the experts. The trial itself will be presided over by a judge, not a jury.

THE ROLE OF COUNSEL

In complex legal cases, the involvement of counsel (barristers or solicitor advocates) becomes essential. Counsel provides specialist legal expertise, advises on legal strategy and represents the health care professional in court proceedings, if necessary. The lawyer and counsel work together closely to ensure a unified approach, leveraging their respective skills and knowledge. Effective coordination and communication between the health care professional, their lawyer and counsel are crucial to presenting a strong case.

CASE CONFERENCES

Conferences are meetings with counsel. They play a vital role in the legal process and are one of the most effective ways of assessing the case. They take place at key stages in the litigation and may be held in person or remotely. Often, experts and others in the legal team also attend.

Counsel is instructed by the legal team and will have been sent papers in advance of a conference. Usually, they talk through the events and seek clarification of the facts and comments from the experts. Such a meeting is a chance to discuss the progress of the case, evaluate evidence and agree on a strategy for the upcoming stages. In sum, these conferences provide an opportunity to address any concerns, seek clarifications and ensure alignment between the health care professional and their legal team.

NOTES

1. https://resolution.nhs.uk/wp-content/uploads/2019/04/NHS-Resolution -Claims-Reporting-Guidelines-Sept-2022-acc-checked.pdf.
2. CPR 32.14.

SECTION **6**

Court

23

Giving evidence in court

Witnesses providing evidence can either be witnesses of fact or expert witnesses.
  The rules relating to the presentation of evidence vary depending on whether
evidence is being given in a coroner's court, a civil court or a criminal court.
  Broadly speaking, evidence can be presented in several ways, including:

- *Documentary evidence*: This includes physical documents, such as policies,
  protocols, medical records and emails that are relevant to the case.
- *Witness statements*: These are written statements from witnesses that state
  their factual accounts of events.
- *Hearsay evidence*: Hearsay evidence is a statement made out of court, which
  is presented in court to prove the truth of its content.
- *Expert evidence*: Expert witnesses can be called to give their opinions on
  technical or scientific matters relevant to the case.
- *Oral evidence*: A witness can give their evidence in person in court.

When presenting evidence in court, it is important to follow the rules of evidence.
These rules determine what is admissible and how it can be presented in court.

FACTUAL WITNESS STATEMENTS

Most medical negligence claims involve and depend on factual evidence, and
it is usual for the health care professionals involved in the incident subject to a
claim to be asked to provide a witness statement. These statements provide factual accounts of events, including:

- The actions taken
- The reasons behind those actions or an explanation of why an alternative
  course of action was not taken
- In certain cases, what could have been done in a hypothetical situation

While the lawyer drafts the statement to ensure that the form and content are
compliant with court rules, the statement is that of the witness and should therefore, as much as possible, be in the words of the witness. The witness should
be completely satisfied with its content and must sign a statement of truth to

DOI: 10.1201/9781003179351-29   119 verify its contents. Should a witness knowingly give false information, they may be found in contempt of court. Thus, it is crucial that the witness has knowledge of or belief in the truthfulness of everything stated in it.

Witnesses of fact should only give factual, not expert (opinion), evidence, although a health care practitioner whose actions have been criticised is allowed to give some opinion evidence.[1] In such circumstances, it should be clear what is factual evidence and what is opinion evidence based on professional judgement and experience. This exception is limited to a health care professional giving evidence regarding their own actions.

If a witness statement contains evidence that is outside the scope of the evidence that the witness is permitted to give orally, the court may strike out the relevant parts of the statement.

EXPERT EVIDENCE

In a medical negligence claim, there are likely to be a number of issues requiring knowledge and expertise not available to a layman. Expert evidence is likely to be required to address issues such as breach of duty, causation of injury and condition and prognosis.

Part 35 of the Civil Procedure Rules deals with expert evidence and the form and content of the reports.

GIVING ORAL EVIDENCE

Not all witnesses of fact or expert witnesses will be required to give oral evidence in court, but if they are, they should remember that first and foremost, their duty is to the court, not the party instructing them.

The GMC's guidance on Good Medical Practice (GMP) (2013), states that doctors must be honest and trustworthy when giving evidence to courts or tribunals and that they must ensure that any evidence given is not false or misleading.

In a subsequent guidance document, 'Giving Evidence in Legal Proceedings', the GMC expands on how doctors should approach giving evidence, whether as a witness of fact (a professional witness) or an expert witness. This guidance clarifies that doctors play an important role in the justice system by contributing evidence both as expert witnesses and witnesses of fact.

Some core principles apply no matter the capacity in which the evidence is given, and such principles apply to health care professionals across the board, such as:

- *The first duty of the witness is to the court.*

  Witnesses are required to uphold the principles of independence, honesty, objectivity and impartiality. Information and insights should be presented based on factual and professional grounds rather than personal opinions. Witnesses should refrain from allowing their personal views or biases about individuals to influence the evidence or advice provided.

- Witnesses should understand their role as a witness throughout the court process.

- Cooperation with case management, including meeting-prescribed times-cales for producing reports and attending conferences, meetings or court hearings, is vital.

- Any report written or evidence provided must be accurate and free from any form of misrepresentation. This entails taking reasonable measures to verify the accuracy of the information presented and ensuring that all relevant information is included.

- Language and terminology should be understandable to those without a medical background. It is essential to provide clear explanations of any abbreviations, medical terms or technical jargon used. Including diagrams with explanatory labels can be helpful.

TIPS FOR GIVING ORAL EVIDENCE

Here are some general tips that health care professionals may find helpful when giving oral evidence:

- *Preparation*

    The health care professional should prepare thoroughly by reviewing relevant medical records, guidelines and other case-related documents so that accurate and well-informed answers to any questions that may arise during the hearing can be given.

    If giving evidence of fact, witnesses should familiarise themselves with their own written statement, as this forms the basis for the questions asked. Witnesses should anticipate areas where evidence may be challenged and con-sider, in advance, how they may respond.

- *Practical points*

    ✓ Know where and when to be at court
    ✓ Arrive on time
    ✓ Dress professionally
    ✓ Bring something to do while waiting, as witnesses may have to wait before giving evidence

- *About mobile phones*

    Mobile phones must be turned off during proceedings

- *Listening to the questions*

    The witness should face and listen to the lawyer who is asking the question and actively listen. If the witness does not understand the question, they should seek clarification before answering.

- *Direct answers to the judge/coroner/jury*

  Witnesses should turn to the judge to answer and see whether the answer is clearly understood. If the judge is making notes, the witness should slow down so that they can record everything accurately, then turn back to the questioning lawyer, ready for the next question.

- *Honesty and objectivity*

  It is important to provide an honest and objective account of what happened, even if it reflects negatively on the witness's actions or decisions or the health care provider. Being truthful and transparent helps establish credibility as a witness.

- *Being clear and concise*

  Simple and clear language must be used when giving evidence. Medical jargon or technical terms that may confuse the judge or jury should be avoided. The witness should be concise, stick to the facts and avoid adding unnecessary detail or personal commentary.

- *Staying calm and composed*

  Giving evidence can be stressful and emotional, but it is important to remain calm and composed throughout the hearing. The witness should listen carefully to each question, take their time when answering and avoid becoming defensive or argumentative.

- *'Sticking to what you know'*

  Witnesses should avoid speculating on issues outside their direct knowledge and refrain from making generalisations.

- *Being respectful and professional*

  Witnesses are representing the medical profession as a whole and should conduct themselves in a respectful and professional manner at all times. They should avoid making personal attacks or comments and focus on providing objective and impartial evidence.

If witnesses are unsure about any aspect of the case or their role as a witness, they should ask their lawyer, who can provide valuable advice on how to effectively present evidence.

NOTE

1. ES v Chesterfield & North Derbyshire Royal Hospital NHS Trust [2003] EW A Civ 1284.

24

What the court and judge are looking for

Medical negligence trials involve complex legal proceedings that aim to determine whether a health care professional breached their duty of care towards a patient, resulting in harm or injury.

As the primary arbiter of justice, the judge plays a crucial role in assessing the merits of the case and arriving at a fair and just outcome. They evaluate the evidence presented by both parties and apply legal principles to determine whether medical negligence has occurred.

During a medical negligence trial, the judge typically looks for expertise, adherence to professional standards, provision of clear and credible evidence and demonstration of empathy and professionalism from medical professionals. Striving for excellence in these areas enhances their credibility, ensuring their testimony is given due weight in the pursuit of justice.

EXPERTISE AND KNOWLEDGE

Whether witnesses of fact or expert witnesses, medical professionals are expected by the judge to demonstrate a high level of expertise and knowledge in their respective fields. This includes a comprehensive understanding of the medical standard of care relevant to the case, procedures and protocols. The judge assesses the qualifications, experience and credibility of the medical professional, considering their education, training, certifications and any specialised knowledge related to the case at hand. They also consider whether the professional possesses the necessary qualifications and expertise to provide an accurate and competent assessment of the case.

THE STANDARD OF CARE

The judge expects medical professionals to uphold and adhere to the standards of their profession. This includes complying with codes of conduct, ethical guidelines and established protocols. The judge looks for evidence of whether the defendant's actions align with accepted medical practices and whether they exercised the required level of skill and care. Therefore, demonstrating a thorough knowledge of professional guidelines and adherence to established protocols is vital to establish credibility in the courtroom.

To determine the standard of care, the judge relies on expert witnesses who testify about the acceptable practices within the relevant field. These experts compare the defendant's actions with those of their peers and help the judge assess whether the defendant deviated from the accepted practice.

BREACH OF DUTY

The judge closely examines whether the health care professional has breached their duty of care owed to the patient. A breach occurs when the professional fails to meet the standard of care established. The judge considers various factors, such as the circumstances surrounding the case, available resources, patient history and any applicable guidelines or protocols.

To establish a breach of duty, the judge may evaluate evidence, including medical records, witness testimonies, expert opinions and any relevant documentation. It is essential for the judge to understand the context in which the medical professional made decisions or took actions that may have led to harm or injury to the patient.

CAUSATION

In a medical negligence trial, establishing causation is crucial. The judge seeks to determine whether the defendant's breach of duty directly caused the harm or injury suffered by the patient. This requires careful analysis of the evidence presented during the trial. The judge relies on medical expert testimony to establish the link between the defendant's actions and the patient's negative outcome.

Medical experts may use scientific research, medical literature and their professional experience to demonstrate how the defendant's breach of duty directly caused or contributed to the patient's harm. The judge considers the strength and reliability of the evidence provided to assess the causal relationship between the defendant's actions and the patient's adverse outcome.

COMMUNICATION AND DOCUMENTATION

The judge also evaluates the communication and documentation practices of medical professionals. Effective communication between medical professionals and patients is vital to ensure informed consent, proper diagnosis and accurate treatment. The judge assesses whether the defendant adequately communicated the risks, benefits and alternatives to the patient, allowing them to make informed decisions.

Moreover, the judge considers the quality of documentation maintained by the defendant. Accurate and comprehensive documentation assists in establishing the chronology of events, treatment plans and any deviations from standard practices. The judge may evaluate medical records, progress notes and other relevant documents to determine the defendant's adherence to proper documentation practices.

PROVISION OF CLEAR AND CREDIBLE EVIDENCE

The judge relies on medical professionals, whether witnesses of fact or expert witnesses, to provide clear and credible evidence to support their testimony. This may involve explaining medical procedures, diagnoses and treatment plans in a manner that can be easily understood by the court. The judge expects medical professionals to present medical records, test results and other relevant documentation that supports their opinions. Furthermore, the judge pays close attention to the consistency and reliability of the medical professional's testimony and the coherence of their explanations, ensuring they can withstand cross-examination.

IMPARTIALITY AND OBJECTIVITY

The judge expects medical professionals to maintain impartiality and objectivity throughout the trial. While they may have an opinion on the matter at hand, medical professionals must present their testimony in an unbiased and objective manner. The judge evaluates whether the medical professionals have appropriately reviewed all relevant information, considered alternative hypotheses and arrived at their conclusions based on sound medical reasoning. It is crucial for medical professionals to avoid any appearance of bias or advocacy for either party, as this may undermine their credibility and the fairness of the trial.

EMPATHY AND PROFESSIONALISM

The judge appreciates medical professionals who demonstrate empathy and professionalism towards the claimant, defendant and their respective legal teams.

Medical negligence cases involve individuals who have suffered harm, and the judge expects medical professionals to exhibit sensitivity and understanding when providing their testimonies.

Maintaining a professional demeanour, answering questions clearly and patiently, and displaying respectful behaviour towards all involved contribute to the overall perception of the medical professional's credibility and integrity.

THE DOWNSIDE OF A CONFRONTATIONAL ATTITUDE

While the adversarial nature of a trial can lead witnesses to adopt a confrontational attitude when giving evidence, this can have several downsides that may undermine their effectiveness. For example:

- *Loss of credibility*

  A confrontational demeanour can make a witness appear defensive, aggressive or evasive, which can lead to a loss of credibility in the eyes of the judge and opposing counsel. It may create the impression that the witness is attempting to hide something or is not being entirely truthful, even if that is not the case. In turn, this can weaken the overall impact of their testimony.

- *Emotional bias*

  A confrontational approach can trigger emotional responses, and a witness who is confrontational risks escalating tensions and allowing emotions to cloud their judgement, potentially diverting attention from the merits of the case.

- *Judge perception*

  A confrontational attitude by a witness can alienate the judge and create a negative impression. The judge may find a confrontational attitude frustrating and may interpret confrontational behaviour as arrogance, lack of cooperation or an attempt to manipulate or disrupt the proceedings. Such perceptions can significantly influence their perception of the witnesses' professionalism, credibility and, ultimately, their evaluation of the evidence and their decision-making process.

Maintaining a calm, composed and cooperative demeanour is generally more advantageous, as it enhances credibility, fosters a positive perception of the witness and allows the evidence to be evaluated objectively.

REMORSE, REFLECTION, HONESTY AND INTEGRITY

Demonstrating genuine remorse, reflection, honesty and integrity helps to establish and maintain trust and credibility with the court and all parties involved in the trial. It directly impacts the perception of the medical professional's character and intentions.

When the witness shows remorse and takes responsibility for any mistakes or errors, it can foster an atmosphere of honesty and integrity, enhancing their credibility and allowing for a more objective evaluation of the case.

Demonstrating reflection and being honest about any errors reflect a commitment to ethical conduct and professionalism and can foster an atmosphere of honesty and integrity. It enhances credibility, helps to counter any negative perceptions and reinforces the notion that the medical professional is concerned about the patient's well-being. This can have a significant impact on the perception of their commitment to patient care and likewise allows for a more objective evaluation of the case.

25

Handling cross-examination

Cross-examination is a pivotal part of a trial, serving as a crucial tool for lawyers to challenge witnesses' credibility and expose weaknesses in their testimony. A skilful cross-examination can sway the mind of the judge, reveal the truth and ultimately determine the outcome of the trial.

For a medical professional, being called as a witness – whether a witness of fact or an expert witness – in a trial can be an intimidating experience, particularly when facing cross-examination. However, with the right mindset and preparation, witnesses can effectively navigate the process, present their evidence with confidence and ensure that their testimony remains credible, consistent and persuasive.

WHAT IS CROSS-EXAMINATION?

Cross-examination plays a significant role in the adversarial legal system, allowing for a thorough examination of the evidence and witnesses in pursuit of justice. It is a legal process that occurs during a trial where one party's counsel questions a witness from the other side. It is an opportunity for counsel to challenge the witness's testimony and credibility and the evidence presented by the opposing party. The purpose of cross-examination is to elicit information that may weaken the witness's testimony, expose inconsistencies or biases or present an alternative interpretation of the events in question.

Cross-examination generally allows for a wide range of questions that are relevant to the case. Through cross-examination, counsel aims to:

- *Undermine the witness's credibility*: This will highlight inconsistencies in their testimony and previous statements or identify biases, prejudices or motives that may affect their reliability.

- *Test the witness's knowledge*: Cross-examination allows counsel to test the witness's knowledge, understanding and memory of events. They may post specific questions to challenge the witness's recollection or to expose any gaps or errors in their evidence.

DOI: 10.1201/9781003179351-31

- *Contradict or challenge the witness's account*: Counsel may present evidence or ask questions that contradict the witness's version of events, challenging their credibility and casting doubt on the accuracy of their evidence.

- *Present alternative interpretations*: Cross-examination provides an opportunity for counsel to introduce alternative theories or explanations for evidence presented by the witnesses. This can help undermine the opposing party's case and provide support for counsel's own arguments.

- *Strengthen their party's case*: Through cross-examination, counsel can elicit admissions from the witness that support their own case or weaken the opposing party's position.

Cross-examination is subject to certain rules and guidelines. Counsel must frame their questions in a manner that adheres to the rules of evidence and the court's guidelines. Questions related to a witness's character are permitted if it is relevant to their credibility. Counsel must also be mindful of maintaining a respectful and professional demeanour towards the witnesses, the court and the jury.

The purpose of cross-examination is not to harass, intimidate or oppress the witness but to rigorously test their testimony and bring out the truth. The court has the authority to intervene and control the conduct of cross-examination to maintain fairness in the proceedings.

PREPARING FOR CROSS-EXAMINATION

Reviewing and familiarising themselves with their previous statements will help the witness ensure that their testimony aligns with previous accounts.

The witness should thoroughly understand the facts, evidence and legal issues in the case and should carefully review all of the evidence in the case – in particular, medical records, formal court documents, such as the particulars of claim, and any written evidence that the parties have exchanged.

Identifying the strengths and weaknesses of the case and the opposing party's case will make it easier for the witness to anticipate their line of attack and should enable the witness to think about how they may respond to questions from counsel.

THE ART OF CROSS-EXAMINATION

Counsel are highly trained in the art of cross-examination. They use key techniques throughout the trial, such as:

- Using questions that require more than a simple 'yes' or 'no' response: This gives the witness the opportunity to explain themselves but may also uncover additional information or reveal inconsistencies in the testimonies.

- Using short and clear questions: Concise, focused and easy-to-understand questions reduce the opportunity for the witness to evade or confuse the issue at hand.

- Avoiding compound questions that address multiple issues simultaneously: This isolates each point of contention and elicits clear and precise responses.

- Building a theme: Developing a coherent theme or theory of the case guides their line of questioning. Using each question to build on previous answers establishes a consistent narrative that supports their argument.

While leading questions are not usually permitted in evidence-in-chief (the initial questioning of one's own witnesses), they are generally permissible during cross-examination.

Counsel actively listens by paying close attention to the witness's responses, body language and vocal cues. They then use their answers as opportunities to ask follow-up questions or highlight contradictions.

HANDLING CROSS-EXAMINATION

When handling cross-examination, the witness should:

- *Listen carefully*: Pay close attention to each question posed by the opposing counsel. The witness should not rush or interrupt during their questioning.

- *Clarify when necessary*: If a question is unclear or ambiguous, the witness should politely request clarification before responding and not assume the meaning or intent of the question.

- *Pause before responding*: The witness should take a moment to gather their thoughts before answering each question to formulate clear and precise responses to avoid impulsive or mistaken answers.

- *Answer directly*: The witness should provide concise, truthful answers, stick to the facts and avoid speculation or guesswork.

- *Not guess or assume*: If the witness does not know the answer to a question, it is acceptable to say, 'I don't know' or 'I don't remember'. The witness should not speculate as it may harm their credibility.

- *Beware of traps*: The witness should be cautious of leading questions or attempts to twist words and listen carefully and address the question asked. They should not volunteer additional information beyond the scope of the question.

- *Maintain eye contact*: A direct gaze towards the judge while answering questions establishes a connection and enhances credibility.

- *Speak clearly and confidently*: The witness should project clearly, enunciate words and speak at a moderate pace. They should be aware of body language and gestures, conveying confidence and honesty.

- *Stay calm and focused*: The witness should maintain a composed and neutral demeanour throughout. They must avoid becoming defensive, argumentative or emotional, as it may undermine their credibility.

RE-EXAMINATION

After cross-examination, the party who called the witness has the opportunity to conduct re-examination.

Re-examination is limited to clarifying any matters raised during cross-examination and addressing any new issues that may have arisen.

26

The role of the expert

Whether an individual is acting as a witness of fact or as an expert witness, they have an overriding duty to the court.

A witness of fact is someone called by the court to give factual evidence based on their personal observations and first-hand knowledge of the events or circumstances related to the case. In a medical negligence trial, factual witness evidence is often provided by the patient and/or their family or friends, the doctor treating the patient and any other health care professionals involved in their care. These witnesses testify about what they saw, heard or experienced and any other relevant details pertaining to the case.

Witnesses of fact are distinct from expert witnesses. Witnesses of fact primarily provide factual information based on their personal observations. By contrast, expert witnesses are individuals with specialist knowledge and expertise in a particular field, who provide professional opinions on the standard of care provided and the cause of any harm suffered.

THE EXPERT WITNESS

> The court invariably needs and invariably depends upon the help it receives from experts in this field. The court has no expertise of its own, other than legal expertise ... The expert advises, but the judge decides. The judge decides on the evidence ... There is, however, no rule that the judge suspends judicial belief simply because the evidence is given by an expert.[1]

An expert witness, also known as a medicolegal expert, is an individual who is qualified and has thorough knowledge or experience to provide an opinion on a particular issue(s) to the court. The expert witness must demonstrate a 'medicolegal mind', which involves applying the correct legal tests to the issues.

An expert witness can be appointed by either the claimant or the defendant, by the parties jointly or, in some instances, directly by the court. They are instructed to comment on the facts using their expertise and medical opinion. Their main

DOI: 10.1201/9781003179351-32

role is to assist the court by providing an impartial medical opinion, regardless of the fact that their fees are paid by those instructing them.

Except in very rare cases, the expert witness is independent and would not have had any dealings with the patient prior to being instructed as part of the legal proceedings. They are required to declare any conflicts of interest at the earliest opportunity.

Expert witnesses do not require formal training to be instructed; however, they are required to comply with the Civil Procedure Rules, particularly Rule 35, which considers the role of experts and the evidence they provide. Experts should understand the importance of their duties to the court and the potential consequences if they fail in them.[2]

The expert witness's evidence can aid the court in reaching a decision about the case, which highlights why it is essential that they provide evidence based on their knowledge/expertise only, are honest and act impartially.

In Jones v Kaney,[3] the Supreme Court clarified that experts do not have the benefit of immunity and can be sued for professional negligence.

THE WITNESS OF FACT

When called to give evidence as a factual witness, first and foremost, the health care professional's role is to present the facts as they experienced or witnessed them, without offering expert opinions or interpretations.

The purpose of having witnesses of fact is to present the court with witness accounts and objective information that can help establish the facts surrounding the alleged negligence. The testimonies can provide critical evidence that supports or contradicts the claims made by the claimant and/or the defendant.

The witness of fact is an ordinary witness; therefore, a health care professional called as a witness in this capacity is expected to act and be treated the same as any other member of the public summoned to attend the court. Thus, they can claim expenses incurred in attending the court.

When a health care professional is called as a factual witness in a medical negligence trial, they may be asked to testify about various aspects of the case, including:

- *Treatment details*

  They may provide a detailed account of the treatment or procedure that was performed, including the specific actions taken, medications administered and any complications that occurred.

- *Patient history*

  They may provide information about the patient's history, pre-existing conditions or any relevant factors that may have influenced the treatment decisions.

- *Communication*

  They may testify about the conversations or discussions that took place between themselves, the patient and other medical staff involved in the care. This can include discussions of potential risks, alternative treatment options or any other relevant information.

- *Documentation*

  They may be asked to review and authenticate medical records, charts or other relevant documents related to the case.

- *Policies or protocols*

  The witness may provide insight into the standard policies or protocols in place, whether these were followed in the case in question and, if not, why they were not.

As the witness of fact providing evidence, the health care professional may be asked to provide the court with evidence of what happened, including clinical findings and observations, and their thoughts during the time in question, such as the reasoning behind the treatment provided.

The witness of fact's evidence must be factual, clear and honest. Questions must be answered truthfully and accurately.

The GMP guidance, published by the GMC, outlines the duties of a doctor registered with the GMC. It highlights key recommendations to doctors who are witnesses of fact, in summary:

- Be honest and trustworthy and avoid being misleading when giving evidence.
- Cooperate with formal inquiries and complaints procedures.
- Make clear the limits of your competence and knowledge.

WHEN CAN A WITNESS OF FACT GIVE OPINION EVIDENCE?

A witness of fact should usually only give evidence of fact. They should not give expert or opinion evidence. This is because a factual witness has no experience in giving expert evidence and no knowledge of the requirements for giving expert evidence. Furthermore, a witness of fact is rarely independent.[4]

A witness of fact can, however, provide opinion evidence on issues in a case *personally perceived by him*.[5] For example:

- *Personal impressions or reactions*

  Witnesses of fact can provide their opinions about their personal impressions or reactions to a situation. For instance, they may express their opinion about someone's behaviour, demeanour or emotional state based on what they observed.

- *Estimations*

  Witnesses of fact may provide opinions regarding, for example, timings that they perceived during an event.

- *Identification*

  Witnesses of fact may offer their opinions about recognising a specific individual or object based on prior knowledge.

- *Common knowledge or everyday matters*

  Witnesses of fact can provide opinions on matters that fall within common knowledge or everyday experiences. This may include expressing opinions about whether the ward was busy, staffing levels or general knowledge about a particular subject.

If the witness of fact strays into giving expert evidence, an application may be made to the court to strike out their evidence.

In a medical negligence case, the health care professional who is a defendant may wish to justify their actions by drawing upon their professional experience. Is that permissible?

In DN v LB Greenwich,[6] the court found that the evidence given by a psychologist in their capacity as a lay witness was admissible, noting that:

> It very often happens in professional negligence cases that a defendant will give evidence to a judge which constitutes the reason why he considers his conduct did not fall below the standard of care reasonable to be expected of him. He may do this by reference to the professional literature that was reasonable available to him as a busy practitioner or by reference to reasonable limits of his professional experience; or he may seek to rebut, as one professional man to another, the criticisms made of him by the claimant's expert(s). Such evidence is common, and it is certainly admissible.

However, the court acknowledged that in these circumstances, the defendant's evidence may lack the objectivity of an independent expert, going to the cogency of the evidence rather than its admissibility. Thus, it did not have the same standing as evidence given by an independent expert. Statements of opinion on matters outside the health care professional's direct experience, arguments and gratuitous comments are inadmissible, as they are for the court to decide.

Health care professionals who are witnesses of fact may therefore give opinion evidence that is reasonably related to the facts within their knowledge and relevant comments based on their own professional experience.

Witnesses of fact should not, however, be advocates, provide submissions[7] or give contentious commentary on documents.[8] They should not attempt to usurp the role of the judge.[9]

The following cases illustrate what witnesses of fact should avoid:

- **YJB Port Ltd v M&A Pharmachem Ltd & another [2021] EWHC 42 (Ch)**

The judge heavily criticised the evidence provided by both the witnesses of fact and expert witnesses. Evidence of fact was found to be of little assistance and comprised largely the witness's analysis and commentary on documents. The witness was not an expert witness and therefore should have avoided providing his opinion.

- **Ceviz v Frawley & another [2021] EWHC 8 (Ch)**

The judge criticised the evidence of a witness of fact. The court found that the witness statement provided did not reflect the individual's opinion but rather the writer's opinion. Furthermore, the statement included comments and commentary, which should have been omitted.

Notably, for the witnesses of fact, the judge highlighted that 'witness statements are for the giving of evidence, not for arguing the case, making points against the opponent or providing commentary on documents'.

- **E.D and F. Man Liquid Products Limited v Patel [2002] 1706 EWHC (QB)**

The witness statement in this case was criticised for providing excessive opinions and comments on the law.

NOTES

1. Re B (Care: Expert Witnesses) [1996] 1 FLR 667.
2. Thimmaya v Lancashire NHS Foundation Trust [2020] 1 WLUK 437.
3. [2011] UKSC 13.
4. Multiplex Constructions (UK) Limited -v- Cleveland Bridge UK Limited [2008] EWHC 2220(TCC).
5. s. 3(2) of the Civil Evidence Act 1972.
6. [2004] EWCA Civ 1659.
7. E.D and F. Man Liquid Products Limited v Patel [2002] 1706 EWHC (QB); Miller v AIG Europe Ltd *(15 January 2016).
8. Kaupthing Singer & Friedlander Ltd (in administration) v. UBS AG [2014] EWHC 2450 (Comm).
9. Rock Nominees v RCO Holdings [2003] EWHC 936 (CH).

27

Who will the court believe?

Many, if not most, medical negligence cases that get to trial rest on issues of fact rather than issues of law.

The court's role is to objectively assess the evidence presented and determine the facts of the case. The court does not have a predetermined bias or preference for either the claimant or the defendant.

In every case, there are some facts that are agreed upon. For example, the parties may agree that the claimant was a patient of the defendant and that the defendant provided care to the claimant on a particular date at a particular hospital.

Some facts, while not agreed, do not depend on memory and are incontrovertible. They may appear in documents, or there may be other evidence, such as photographs or videos.

However, some facts are strongly in dispute. The judge will need to make a finding of fact, but who should the court believe?

Each case is unique, and the court's decision will depend on the specific facts and circumstances presented during the trial. The judge's role is to weigh the evidence objectively and make a determination based on the balance of probabilities.

THE GESTMIN PRINCIPLES

In the case of Gestmin SGPS S.A. v Credit Suisse,[1] the court was tasked with evaluating the evidence of numerous witnesses concerning various events that took place over a number of years. In an interesting judgement, the judge considered the psychology of recollection, psychological research and the fallibility of human memory. Although they are specific to that case, they have been influential in subsequent cases and provide guidance on how courts should approach witness testimony. Here are the key principles:

- *Human memory is fallible.*

  The court recognises that human memory is not infallible and can be influenced by various factors, such as the passage of time, perception and individual perspectives and biases. This principle acknowledges that witnesses may

 DOI: 10.1201/9781003179351-33

not accurately recall events and emphasises caution when relying solely on memory.

- *Memory is an active reconstructive process.*

  The court acknowledges that memory is a reconstructive process rather than a verbatim recording of events. Witnesses often (subconsciously) fill in gaps in their memory with assumptions, speculation or information from external sources. The court should be aware of this and consider the limitations of memory when assessing witness evidence.

- *Documentation and contemporaneous records.*

  The court emphasises the importance of contemporaneous documents and records in corroborating or contradicting witness testimony. Such documents provide a more reliable and accurate account of events, reducing the fallibility of memory.

- *Oral evidence is not always reliable.*

  The court recognises that oral evidence, including witness testimony, can be subject to errors, distortions or misrepresentations. The court should not rely solely on oral evidence if there are other objective sources of information available.

- *Witness credibility should be assessed.*

  The court should assess the credibility of witnesses by considering the consistency of their evidence with the documents and other evidence, their demeanour, the inherent probability or improbability of their account and the extent to which their evidence is corroborated by other evidence.

  The Gestmin principles underline the need for courts to approach witness evidence with caution, recognising the limitations of memory and the potential for biases or errors. They emphasise the importance of relying on contemporaneous documents and objective evidence when available to establish a more accurate account of events.

ASSESSING CREDIBILITY

Credibility is not the same as honesty. It is possible for two witnesses to provide honest testimonies about the same events, yet one or both of them may be completely mistaken. In such cases, rather than assuming one witness is dishonest, the judge endeavours to find a resolution that avoids unnecessary controversy and seeks to identify a plausible explanation for the apparent conflict between the differing accounts.

In Synclair v East Lancashire Hospital NHS Trust,[2] the claimant told a doctor that his surgical stoma had changed colour. A medical note, written by a different junior doctor, said 'stoma normal colour'. The claimant was adamant that this junior doctor had not been present when he told the first about the colour change. The judge concluded that there was no necessary inconsistency if the junior doctor was not present when the claimant told the doctor about the colour change.

The judge needs to consider a number of issues when deciding which witness to believe.

In the case of Onassis v Vergottis,[3] Lord Pearce suggested that when considering witness credibility, it would be appropriate to consider the following questions:

- Is this witness a truthful or untruthful person?
- Is the witness telling the truth on this issue?
- Is the witness remembering correctly?
- Is the witness mistaken?

In the case of McAllister v Campbell,[4] the court provided guidance on how credibility is assessed. The case was a personal injury claim, and the court outlined several factors that judges should consider when evaluating witness credibility, such as:

- *Consistency and coherence of evidence*

  The court should assess whether the witness's evidence is consistent and coherent, both internally and when compared with other evidence presented. Any inconsistencies or contradictions may impact the witness's credibility.

- *Corroboration and supporting evidence*

  The court should consider whether the witness's evidence is corroborated by other witnesses or supported by the objective evidence, such as documents or physical evidence. Corroborative evidence can strengthen a witness's testimony.

  In Grimstone v Epson & St Helier University Hospitals NHS Trust, the resolution of an evidential dispute relied on the use of contemporaneous records. The dispute centred around the content of a consultation between the claimant and her doctor regarding a surgical procedure. The doctor, despite not recalling the specifics of the consultation, provided evidence regarding his usual practice, which was supported by corroborative medical records. The claimant presented her own recollection of events, which was different from the doctor's account. Ultimately, the court favoured the records and the doctor's evidence of his consistent practice.

Conversely, in Hughes v Royal United Hospital Bath NHS Trust,[5] the claimant alleged surgical negligence. The court found that the surgeon's evidence lacked credibility and was inconsistent with the other evidence presented. The judge criticised the surgeon's approach to the case, noting that his evidence contained contradictions and that he had not provided a convincing explanation for certain decisions and actions taken during the surgery. The judge also highlighted instances where the surgeon's account conflicted with the contemporaneous medical records and other witness testimony. In its judgement, the court ultimately rejected the surgeon's version of events and found for the claimant. The court's critical assessment of the surgeon played a significant role in reaching this conclusion.

- *Plausibility and inherent probability*

The court should assess the plausibility and inherent probability of the witness's evidence in the context of the case. If the witness's testimony seems implausible or highly improbable, it may impact their credibility.

In the case of Caldero Trading v Beppler & Jacobson Ltd,[6] the court recognised that due to the lack of pertinent documentation, it was necessary to consider the broader context and probabilities surrounding the agreement. An assessment of 'overall commercial probabilities' played a vital role in determining the terms of the contract in question.

- *Motive and interest*

The court should examine any motives or interests that the witness may have in the outcome of the case. Personal biases or conflicts of interest can affect the witness's credibility and should be taken into account.

- *Demeanour and manner of the witness*

The court should observe the demeanour and manner of the witness during their testimony, including their behaviour, attitude and responses. This can provide insights into their credibility and reliability.

In Grimstone, the claimant's course of action, had she received the advice she alleged the doctor negligently failed to provide, became a critical question. However, during cross-examination, the claimant refused to disclose whether she would have chosen a specific course of action if she had been informed that it was the optimal option. Consequently, the judge concluded that there was no doubt that she would have followed the recommended advice.

That said, while a witness's demeanour can carry weight, it is a vague concept that judges approach cautiously. Understandably, emotions can alter a witness's demeanour, and the courts remain mindful of this. Additionally, judges are understandably hesitant to draw conclusions based solely on demeanour when the witness is not a native English speaker or has a cultural background unfamiliar to the judge.

- *Past record and credibility history*

The court may consider the witness's past record and credibility history, including any prior inconsistent statements or previous findings of dishonesty or unreliability. This can influence the court's assessment of their credibility.

Nevertheless, each case is unique, and the court's evaluation of credibility may depend on the specific facts and circumstances presented. The court's role is to assess the credibility of witnesses objectively and make a determination based on the evidence and applicable legal standards.

NOTES

1. [2013] EWCA 3560 (Comm).
2. [2015] EWCA Civ 1283.
3. [1968] 2 Lloyds Rep 403.
4. [2014] NIQB 24.
5. [2020] EWHC 1937 (QB).
6. [2012] EWHC 1609 (Ch).

SECTION 7

Negligence and clinical errors

28

Allegations of negligence

Typically, when the claimant's solicitor submits documents, they contain allegations of negligence. These are what the health care professional is accused of and detail how they breached their duty of care to the patient. Although the precise allegations depend on the circumstances and the speciality, some common themes warrant discussion from a clinical rather than a legal perspective.

WRONG DIAGNOSIS AND DELAYED DIAGNOSIS

A wrong diagnosis is not a breach of duty. We are all human, so we can and we will be wrong at times. The standard required of the health care professional is not that of a super doc or a professor of a specific ailment. Instead, competence should fit within the Bolam test, namely that our conduct reaches the standard of a responsible body of medical opinion.

Take this case, for example. A patient presented with a condition, and the doctor utilised their clinical acumen to make a diagnosis of A.

However, another clinician subsequently made the correct diagnosis of B, and the patient makes a complaint that the first doctor failed to diagnose condition B and instead made the incorrect diagnosis of condition A, thus leading to more attendances, prolonged suffering and harm.

The patient claims that the first doctor was negligent in making a diagnosis of A and that there was a delayed diagnosis of condition B, which resulted in harm.

The key question is whether it was reasonable to make a diagnosis of condition A and whether other clinicians would have made a similar diagnosis. It does not need to be every other clinician but instead a reasonable body of medical opinion. Exactly what this means is a matter of debate. Does 10% of colleagues make up a reasonable body of medical opinion? Does 1%?

In the end, it is mostly whether the medical experts engaged by the claimant and by the defendant feel the conduct was reasonable. Guidelines and evidence in the literature help determine what is reasonable and emphasise the need to follow and to be able to demonstrate the guidelines and evidence-based practice where possible.

When making the judgement as to whether a diagnosis of A was reasonable, the medical experts and the courts will have to use the clinical record to make a determination. If there is not enough information in the record or if the diagnostic rationale is unclear, then this can be a potential weakness.

Causation is also important. With the diagnosis of condition A and then eventually condition B, it must be proven that this delay or misdiagnosis altered the outcome of the patient. The misdiagnosis has to have caused harm. If condition B is untreatable, then even with an earlier diagnosis, the outcome would have been the same; hence, there is no causation for the final harm.

Causation relies on the question 'on the balance of probabilities, but for the alleged breach of duty, would the adverse outcome have occurred?'

UNREASONABLE DELAY IN DIAGNOSIS

In certain scenarios, there is a reasonable and 'allowable' uncertainty in diagnosis. For instance, the patient presented with symptoms and signs consistent with a diagnosis of A. The condition worsened, evolved and failed to respond to treatment. At some stage, the diagnosis of B was made. Although the diagnosis of A was reasonable, the patient complains and litigates, asserting that the diagnosis of B should have been made sooner and that if it had, the outcome would have been better.

In this situation, the court and the experts are required to determine when the diagnosis of B should have been made by a reasonably competent doctor. The longer the delay, the greater the likelihood of breach of duty. It places the experts into a situation where they have to determine how long is too long. Where does the delay in diagnosis become unreasonable and a breach of duty? The symptoms and signs are key, and they will need to be documented clearly to allow the experts and the court to say it was reasonable to stick with diagnosis A at that stage in the clinical course.

The following statements would have to be evaluated: once A fails to resolve and no other diagnosis is considered, then the clinician may be criticised. Once the symptoms and signs inconsistent with a diagnosis of A develop and the clinician fails to consider another diagnosis, such as condition B, then they may be criticised.

The problem with this scenario is that multiple clinicians may be involved. The first clinician made a diagnosis of A, and that was entirely reasonable. That diagnosis was propagated from then on, and no one challenged it or sought any differential diagnoses. So, while the first clinician failed to make the correct diagnosis, no fault lies with them. It is the clinicians down the line who failed to review the condition and the diagnosis who can be criticised. Often in a hospital setting, it is the consultant in overall charge of the patient who faces the blame as captain of the ship, even if they have had no contact with the patient at all. They will have to shoulder the blame, and the patient may have come to harm. Thus, the consultant would have failed in their duty of care.

FAILURE TO CONSIDER

This is a very common allegation of negligence. At its simplest level, a patient presents with a certain condition. The differential diagnosis is x, y and z. Using clinical acumen, the doctor excludes diagnosis y and z and settles on diagnosis x. Treatment commences, but the patient does not get better and indeed worsens. It was eventually found that they have disorder z and thus, they have come to harm.

The patient complains that the doctor made the wrong diagnosis. A reasonable body of medical opinion supports the diagnosis when faced with the symptoms and signs documented.

However, the patient's expert asserts that a reasonable body of medical opinion would have considered not just one diagnosis but also a diagnosis of y and z. Furthermore, when condition x did not improve, the defendant did not consider changing the diagnosis to z.

Indeed, when scrutinising the clinical record, no evidence was found that a diagnosis of z was considered at any stage.

The patient's expert also asserts that had a diagnosis of z been considered, then it is likely that the treatment would have been changed and the patient would not have come to harm.

Given that the clinician's statement mentioned that y and z were considered and then excluded based on their clinical findings, the court must decide whether the doctor did indeed consider the diagnosis and if they did, why they did not act upon it. They do this with the benefit of knowing that the diagnosis was indeed z.

This scenario could have been avoided by clearly documenting the differential diagnosis and explaining in the clinical record why y and z were excluded.

Below is an example of an actual case with similar circumstances:

A 32-year-old man presented to his GP with chest pain. The GP clearly documented that the patient was a non-smoker and had no direct or family history of ischaemic heart disease. The pain was left-sided and did not radiate down the patient's arm. It was worse with inhalation and reproduced to some degree by pressing on the chest. There was no shortness of breath associated with the pain.

A diagnosis of musculoskeletal chest pain was made, and the patient was discharged with appropriate safety netting. 'Unlikely to be cardiac chest pain due to age and nature of the pain. Pain mostly reproduced by chest squeeze', was clearly documented in the clinical record.

However, the man presented to the emergency department 3 days later, and a diagnosis of myocardial infarction was made.

The patient made an allegation of negligence in making the incorrect diagnosis and failing to consider cardiac chest pain. The experts on both sides agreed that the history and examination were consistent with mechanical chest pain and that a reasonable body of GPs would have made a similar diagnosis. The GP had also appropriately safety-netted, and the patient had followed this advice by attending the hospital when the pain worsened.

PROCEDURE NOT COMPLETED TO AN ACCEPTABLE STANDARD

This allegation typically refers to interventional procedures, such as surgery. It is often linked with an allegation surrounding consent.

For example, things go wrong in an operation and the patient claims that the surgeon has breached their duty in carrying out the procedure to an unacceptable level.

In this circumstance, it is difficult to apply the Bolam or Bolitho standard tests for breach of duty. It cannot be said that a detrimental outcome to a surgery would be an accepted standard of care supported by a reasonable body of medical opinion. For example, a post-operative fatal bleed after a hemicolectomy can never be deemed acceptable. However, that does not indicate negligence per se.

There may be a perception that a good surgeon should be able to carry out every procedure without complication, but this is not true. Where the onset of a complication goes over the line to a breach of duty is hard to determine.

Is the surgeon who did not clip an arterial vessel adequately, which resulted in a post-operative bleed, negligent in their technique?

Did the surgeon who undertook a hip replacement, which subsequently became infected, breach their duty in not maintaining asepsis?

These are recognised complications of surgery and can happen without negligence. Thus, individual experts in their fields have to act as detectives to determine whether a complication is due to a substandard level of surgery.

It should be stated that patients cannot consent to negligent treatment, and therefore, if a hip infection occurs because the surgeon has decided to not prepare the skin, then even if infection is on the consent form, it is still a breach of duty that has caused harm.

It is important that all clinicians undertaking interventional procedures keep a record of their complications so they can benchmark themselves against published standards. A regular audit will prove invaluable when demonstrating surgical competence.

For example, if the national total knee replacement infection rate is 1%, then it is to be expected that 1 in 100 patients will develop an infection whoever operates upon them. If, however, a patient develops an infection and the surgeon who has operated on them is found to have a 10% infection rate and has had an investigation into their outcomes as an outlier, then this may have an impact on the perception of breach of duty. This is not evidence per se, as each individual case must be taken in isolation. Nonetheless, all information pertinent to the case may be disclosable.

We are at risk of moving towards the scenario in the USA where high-risk cases are not operated upon for fear of litigation.

Complications are not breaches of duty per se, but they may be. The expert must decide how a complication occurred and whether the standard of surgery was acceptable. In order to facilitate this detective work, they have to assess the evidence, which is the clinical record. Operation notes are vital in this task and need to be thorough and detailed in any case, but all the more so when complications or difficulties arise. The expert needs to understand what was faced, what happened and why in order to formulate an opinion as to the standard of care provided.

Complications will occur, and they are always undesirable. Consent is key when a complication does occur, as is candour. The health care professional must explain to the patient what happened and document it carefully.

FAILURE TO PROVIDE A SAFETY NET

Safety netting is the process of information provision to a patient or their carer about symptoms or signs to look out for and actions to take if their condition fails to improve or changes or if they have further concerns about their health. With the stresses upon health care services, safety netting has become even more important.

A sample case is when a patient sees a doctor and is diagnosed with condition A. Treatment commences, and a follow-up is arranged for 6 months later. The patient attends the emergency department after 4 months because of worsening symptoms. When they attend, they have a 2-month history of symptoms consistent with complication B, which can occur in one in ten cases. Harm has occurred, and the patient alleges a breach of duty in failing to provide a safety net and a failure to communicate and warn of the potential onset of B. Due to the delay in seeking attention, the patient has suffered irreversible harm due to B. Had appropriate safety netting been undertaken, the patient would have been aware of the symptoms of B and would have sought attention earlier. Thus, harm would have been avoided.

There may be a perception that the patient surely would have known to seek attention if they got worse, and it should be incumbent upon them to take responsibility, but that is not an argument that will carry significant weight. The patient has sought care from a professional, and they were reliant upon that professional to advise them. They were reassured that 6 months until their next review was appropriate.

Safety netting is an important aspect of keeping patients safe and should be part of management. Ideally, safety netting should be in verbal and written form, and it should be documented in the clinical record.

FAILURE TO FOLLOW-UP

With the pressures the health care service is facing, more claims are coming through related to administrative failures to organise follow-up appointments in a timely manner. An error may be due to a member of the administrative staff not acting on a request, or it may be related to capacity issues where there is simply no space to see the patient.

In this example, the patient sees a clinician, and a follow-up is planned for 4 months later. The appointment is not made or is delayed, and the patient eventually is seen 12 months later. The patient has come to harm due to the progression of their condition, and they allege a breach of duty.

Clearly, if the clinician requested a follow-up appointment in 4 months, there was a clinical reason for doing so. That reason must have been to avoid harm to the patient. In delaying the follow-up, there was a foreseeable risk of harm to the patient. If the harm does occur, then it is difficult to defend.

Although mitigating circumstances may be taken into consideration, such as the capacity problems within the health service, when it comes to individual cases, courts do not give out 'get out of jail free' cards. Furthermore, the COVID-19 pandemic has seen unprecedented and unavoidable delays in seeing patients. We are yet to see whether the courts will be lenient in these extraordinary circumstances.

If a patient cannot be seen on time, then it is reasonable to expect them to have been triaged to assess risk. If patient A is deemed low risk, then they may be able to wait for a follow-up. Patient B may be at more risk of harm and therefore should be seen sooner. In this circumstance, the organisation has made an effort to manage the risk of harm and ensure equity of care in difficult circumstances. Patient A may still come to harm, but the defence is that there was an effort to triage the patient, and they were deemed to be at low risk of harm. It is not clear whether this will be an adequate defence, but at least an effort was made to mitigate harm.

If there is no attempt at triage and no effort was made to try and keep patients safe in circumstances where the capacity meant that there was no way patients could be seen, then criticism may follow.

Foreseeability can play a role in how the courts view allegations of breach of duty. It was entirely unforeseeable that the COVID-19 pandemic would ensue and that the health care service would effectively collapse. It is entirely foreseeable that delays to surgery and follow-ups due to capacity issues may result in harm, and therefore, it is arguable that the organisation owes a duty of care to all their patients to put steps in place to mitigate and manage that harm.

Once it can be demonstrated that there was a delay in the follow-up, it is incumbent upon the claimant to prove that that delay resulted in harm and that if they were seen as planned, they would have had a better outcome.

DELAY TO SURGERY

Once a decision has been made to proceed to surgery or other intervention, then there is inevitably a delay until treatment. How long a delay is reasonable is debatable. A pathology may progress while waiting for surgery, and in the vast majority of circumstances, the pathology will be entirely reversed. But what if the delay means that there is some residual detriment? Should a patient be allowed to claim for that harm as a direct result of the delay to surgery?

Trusts are balancing capacity and demand, and there will be delays to surgery. This is unavoidable, and it is unreasonable to expect health care organisations to be penalised for this.

The key is that undue delay that results in preventable irreversible harm may represent a breach of duty.

For example, if a listing form is mislaid and the surgery is delayed 6 months longer than was necessary, there may be a reasonable basis for a complaint.

The aim of litigation and compensation is to put the claimant into the position they would have been if the negligence/breach of duty had not occurred. This is impossible for irreversible harm, and so a monetary payout is the substitute. If the harm is resolved by the surgery, albeit delayed, then there is no real prospect of compensation, even though prolonged suffering has been endured.

An expert will have to determine what an undue delay actually means, which is not clear-cut due to different wait times and capacity issues in various health care settings.

FAILURE TO CONSENT

Consent warrants an entire chapter (Chapter 3), as it is a complex issue. Complaints and litigation regarding failure to consent are increasing. Since the pivotal case of Montgomery detailed in an earlier chapter, the issue of consent has come to the fore.

The GMC has recently updated its guidance on consent in 2020.[1] It details seven principles of consent:

- *Principle one*: All patients have the right to be involved in decisions about their treatment and care and to be supported to make informed decisions if they are able.

- *Principle two*: Decision making is an ongoing process focused on meaningful dialogue, in other words, the exchange of relevant information specific to the individual patient.

- *Principle three*: All patients have the right to be listened to and to be given the information they need to make a decision and the time and support they need to understand it.

- *Principle four*: Doctors must try to find out what matters to patients so that they can share relevant information about the benefits and harms of proposed options and reasonable alternatives, including the option to take no action.

- *Principle five*: Doctors must start from the presumption that all adult patients have the capacity to make decisions about their treatment and care. A patient can only be judged to lack the capacity to make a specific decision at a specific time and only after an assessment in line with legal requirements.

- *Principle six*: The choice of treatment or care for patients who lack capacity must be of overall benefit to them, and decisions should be made in consultation with those who are close to them or advocating for them.

- *Principle seven*: Patients whose right to consent is affected by law should be supported to be involved in the decision-making process and to exercise choice if possible.

When the benefits of a procedure are realised, then patients do not complain about the consent process. Thus, in the vast majority of cases, consent is never an issue that causes contention. This has lulled the health care profession into adopting lax processes regarding consent. The Montgomery case has acted as a timely reminder that we need to respect patient autonomy and pay more than lip service to the issue of consent. The 'just sign here' mentality of consent has rightly been relegated to history.

The GMC commissioned work regarding patients' attitudes towards consent and decision making, which produced valuable qualitative findings.[2] Several recommendations for improving communication include:

- Smile, use open body language and be friendly.
- Use simple terminology and speak slowly.
- Be prepared to repeat information.
- Provide reassurance.
- Establish the need for and promote interpreter and translation services.
- Check whether the patient can read or write.
- Employ visual aids in addition to verbal communication.
- Provide information for people to take away, such as leaflets, and offer these in other languages.
- Allow the patient time to ask questions or to raise queries.
- Ask the patient how much they would like the person with them to be involved.
- Provide a written overview of what was discussed in consultations.
- Cater for people with visual and hearing impairments (e.g. audio information, verbalising others' presence and digital signage).

These recommendations are sensible steps to avoid complaints regarding the consent process.

When things go wrong and one of the complications – which might have been theoretical and unlikely to occur – actually manifests, then the consent issue comes to the fore. Evidence has shown that patients' recollection and understanding of medical procedures, risks and complications are often limited, particularly among older individuals. Unsurprisingly, when things go wrong, patients often claim that they were not told of the risks of surgery or any other procedure. In addition, there is a natural tendency to feel that 'it won't happen to me', and the clinician has to try and explain the risks of the procedure in a balanced manner.

The typical situation is that a patient is planned for a procedure. They have a consultation with the clinician undertaking the procedure or their representative, and they sign a consent form. The consent form may have numerous risks on it or very few.

The procedure is carried out, but a complication ensues with a detrimental outcome. The patient then asserts that they did not know the complication could occur; furthermore, if they had been told that the complication/harm could occur, then they would not have had the procedure done.

The clinician is then in a position of stating that the patient was indeed told of the complication and was fully aware of it.

The clinician can use contemporaneous notes to justify their position and point to written comments in the clinical record, such as 'the risk of nerve injury was explained and accepted'; the consent form itself, which may have 'nerve injury' on it; their standard practice of always telling patients about the risks of nerve damage, as evidenced by their witness statement; and any patient information literature provided to the patient.

If all the above are present, then the defendant's case is strengthened. Without any of the above, the court may determine that the specific material risks of nerve injury, as an example, were not discussed with the patient.

The patient may assert that even though the clinician had written the risk of nerve injury in the notes and on the consent form, it was not explained to them in sufficient detail. They may assert that they were never provided with an information leaflet or if they were, they were not told to read it or had the significance of it explained.

Furthermore, the patient may state that they would not have proceeded with the procedure if they had known it could go wrong and cause harm. This is key in order to prove causation. In such a case, the claimant must show that the alleged breach of duty would have affected their outcome. In consent cases, this is usually a decision not to proceed, thus resulting in the avoidance of all the procedure-related harm.

The patient before the procedure, when the likelihood of harm is very low, is different from the patient once the harm has occurred. The court may seek to determine what a reasonable patient would have done in the same circumstances. They will assess the claimant's condition/morbidity and the risk/benefit profile of the intended procedure and try to determine whether they would have indeed refused surgery.

Consent is a vital part of caring for patients. There is a real risk of a miscarriage of justice for patients by not accepting liability when they genuinely were not told of a potential complication. On the other hand, there is also a risk of the opposite when patients were genuinely told about the possible complications but failed to appreciate them. Improving the consent process will serve to protect from both eventualities.

REFERENCES

1. Sherlock A., & Brownie, S. (2014). Patients' recollection and understanding of informed consent: A literature review. *ANZ J Surg* 84, 207–210.
2. Attitudes Towards Consent And Decision Making, Prepared for the General Medical Council by Ipsos MORI, September 2018; https://www.gmc-uk.org/-/media/gmc-site-images/about/attitudes-towards-consent-and-decision-making.pdf?la=en&hash=41B151991F8E61424CE95A8887AADC97CD9761D3] https://www.gmc-uk.org/ethical-guidance/ethical-guidance-for-doctors/decision-making-and-consent.

29

Never events

According to the NHS, '*Never Events are defined as Serious Incidents that are wholly preventable because guidance or safety recommendations that provide strong systemic protective barriers are available at a national level and should have been implemented by all healthcare providers*'.[1]

A never event is called such because these events or errors are not meant to happen. A never event may result in death or permanent disability for a patient and is preventable. For example, surgery performed on the wrong part of the body, surgery performed on the wrong person, leaving surgical instruments inside the body after surgery, giving blood products to the wrong patient and having equipment fall on patients during surgery qualify as never events.

Although technically, never events should not happen, they do and with alarming frequency. According to one study, the NHS paid out on approximately 800 successful never event claims between 2004 and 2014 in surgical specialities alone.[2] The NHS has a list of never events that is updated every few years to ensure that doctors and health care personnel are informed of events that, should they occur, would lead to serious consequences and thus require reporting to the proper administration.[3]

According to the NHS, to qualify as a never event, a situation must fulfil certain criteria, such as:

- The event has to be wholly preventable when following the national guidance or safety recommendations.
- All never events have the *potential* to create serious patient harm or death.
- There are reports of the event happening in the past.
- All never events are clearly defined and easily recognised.[4]

DOI: 10.1201/9781003179351-36

The causes that usually lead to never events and patient harm are multifaceted and interlaced with system failures. The most common never events and their possible causes are:[3]

- *Surgical*
  - ✓ Wrong-site surgery or wrong implant/prosthesis: These errors may occur when there is inadequate or inaccurate preoperative information, poor intraoperative communication or lack of appropriate or consistent use of a process to verify the correct anatomical site.
  - ✓ Retained foreign object post-procedure: Such mistakes are made by the surgical team.
  - ✓ Extracting the wrong tooth: This is a recent addition to the never events list. This can occur when the patient is referred and the surgeon fails to take an appropriate history or perform an oral examination.

- *Medication*
  - ✓ Mis-selection of a strong potassium solution, an overdose of insulin due to abbreviations or the incorrect device, an overdose of methotrexate for non-cancer treatment or mis-selection of high-strength midazolam during conscious sedation: these can occur due to wrong medication prescriptions; or mistaken syringe sizes during administration; mix-ups in packaging, labelling or storage; incorrect mixture of medications, etc.
  - ✓ Administration of medication by the wrong route: Usually due to lack of knowledge of the doctor, a mistake in writing or reading a prescription or miscommunication between seniors and juniors.

- *Mental health*
  - ✓ Failure to install a functional collapsible shower or curtain rails: This is due to hospital authority oversight.

- *General*
  - ✓ Falls from poorly restricted windows, chest or neck entrapment in bed rails or scalding of patients. Failing to identify potential patients at risk of harm may also result in harm and allegations of breach of duty. In the Withers case in 2016, the hospital was found responsible after they failed to remove a risky ladder from a chimney. Mr Withers, who was a mental health patient, climbed up it and fell to his death.[5] It is usually the organisations that have to face these claims rather than the clinician. However, the clinician may have to answer for failing to identify a high-risk person when they fall or accidentally injure themselves.
  - ✓ Transfusion or transplantation of ABO-incompatible blood components or organs.
  - ✓ Misplaced naso- or oro-gastric tubes.
  - ✓ Unintentional connection of a patient requiring oxygen to an air flowmeter.

Never event claims are hard to defend because they should never happen, and processes are usually in place to stop them happening. The organisation and the working clinicians have to fail in their professional duties for these to occur, which is tantamount to admitting negligence.

Although at a glance, these mistakes seem easy enough to avoid, they occur at persistent and alarming rates. Between 1 April 2021 and 28 February 2022, 407 serious incidents were reported.[6] Among them, 379 match the criteria of never events. Twenty-eight incidents did not match the criteria but were serious events.[7]

According to several authors, including Burnett, Norris and Flin, several systemic factors are at work behind the occurrence of never events.[8] For example, workspace and environmental factors, such as changing the operation theatre setting to an unfamiliar layout, can mean the surgical team struggles to perform. This is often compounded by poor planning, leading to instrument unavailability, which is a common contributing factor in never events. In fact, in one out of seven surgical procedures, there is an equipment problem.[9]

Many factors can contribute to the occurrence of a never event, including but not limited to different norms in a different hospital leading to miscommunication through written and computerised notes or miscommunication in the details of a prosthesis. Definite errors on the health provider's part, such as failure to follow protocol, failure to read the notes/charts of the patient and failure to properly mark the surgical site, may also cause never events.

A case of wrong-site surgery shows how mistakes can accumulate and escalate. A patient was admitted for a right far lateral L3/4 microdiscectomy. Before the surgery, the surgical site was marked by the SpR with a non-permanent marker. The consultant arrived at the theatre late and was not present for the marking. During the pre-surgical preparation, the mark washed off, and the surgeon placed a new one and proceeded to cut. Unfortunately, the surgeon operated on the wrong side, a clear never event.[8] Similarly, there have been cases where the wrong kidney of a patient was removed.[10]

James Reason explained with his Swiss cheese model that, despite having multiple levels of protection against such mistakes, such as doctors, nurses, pharmacists and administrative controls all utilising checklists, the failures keep happening.[11] In the model, safety barriers are represented by slices of cheese. These barriers are not solid and impenetrable like true walls of cheese but rather have holes, hence the term Swiss cheese. While each slice has its unique pattern of holes, they all have the same general shape: that of a triangle with the point facing downwards. Occasionally, the holes align in such a way that they allow an error to pass through the whole slice of cheese, resulting in harm.

In themselves, these errors are harmless; they are not strong enough to cause an incident on their own. However, if several errors happen at once and it so happens that the holes in several slices also align during that period, then an incident or accident potentially resulting in harm can result.

With the Swiss cheese model, it is less about preventing these mistakes than making sure that when one does occur, there is another layer to stand in its way and stop it from causing harm.

Apart from the fact that these events should never happen, there is another purpose for declaring an error as a never event, which is the post-event protocol. When a never event occurs, it must be immediately notified to the Strategic Executive Information System (StEIS) and the National Reporting and Learning System (NRLS).[3] Both reports must mention the event as a never event, even if unsure at the moment. Afterwards, if necessary, the status of the incident in the StEIS report can be amended. Some events that are no longer considered a never event, such as wrong-level spine surgery, do not have to be reported. But events that qualify should be reported as soon as they are discovered, even if the incident took place many years prior.

Hospital boards or organisational leaders must ensure a systematic investigation takes place following a never event. The outcome of the investigation should be a clear, concise report that identifies the root causes, contributory causes and immediate causes, with recommendations for immediate, short-term and long-term actions.

Organisations must also take responsibility for addressing any issues arising from never events as soon as possible, including implementing measures to prevent future occurrences. The commissioner's annual report and the provider's quality accounts should also have the details of the never event, along with the steps taken to prevent it

Failure to report a never event is unacceptable and signals a culture of organisational safety failures. If failing to report a never event was unintentional, the organisational lead will need to investigate the situation and find the cause of the failure. If it was deliberate, the staff will be considered to have seriously failed their duty, and the organisation will be considered to have made a breach of CQC requirements.[12]

NATIONAL HEALTH SERVICE IMPROVEMENTS FOR NEVER EVENTS

The NHS Patient Safety Strategy was implemented in 2019 to prevent serious adverse events such as never events.[13] The strategy has been updated annually since to better suit the needs of the patients and systems and to make sure patients are protected from avoidable harm and experience safe care every time they interact with the health and care system. The strategy started with a few goals, such as reducing harm caused by medicines, including reducing prescribing errors and improving medicines adherence; reducing health care-associated infections; reducing sepsis deaths; improving mother and baby care; preventing suicide and self-harm in mental health settings; and improving elderly patient care.

Each year, the safety strategies are improved upon and added to. For example, in 2021, the following safety care strategies were implemented:

1. The Patient Safety Specialists Initiative was launched in 2021 with the goal of employing specialists who can defend patients' safety and oversee the various

programmes and systems to ensure all safety measures are being maintained. Currently, there are 700 individuals at NHS trusts and CCGs who fulfil this role.

2. The Learn from Patient Safety Events (LFPSE) service was launched as the NHS record system for patient safety events. Both local risk management organisations are able to record safety events in LFPSE online, so the data is more diverse, allowing for better preventive planning.

3. The framework for patient safety was updated, providing guidance for patients, families and carers on how to ensure their own safety as well as the staff's.

4. The NHS also published the patient safety syllabus for all NHS staff to have the appropriate knowledge to ensure best patient care and safety.

5. The NHS published a Patient Safety Incident Response Framework website, which establishes a standard protocol for organisational responses to patient safety incidents and details regarding patient safety investigations.

Thus, the NHS is taking steps to ensure that never events truly become never events. Still, as seen in the case reports, standard protocols and robust changes in communication processes, hospital management and systemic investigations are needed to effectively prevent never events.

REFERENCES

1. Improvement NHS. (2018). *Never events policy and framework*. Revised January 2018.
2. Ford, K. E., & Cooper, L. R. (2018). Learning from lawsuits: Ten-years of NHS litigation authority claims against 11 surgical specialities in England. *The Surgeon*, 16(1), 27–35.
3. Improvement NHS. (2018). *Revised never events policy and framework*. Retrieved February 2021, from https://improvement.nhs.uk/documents /2265/Revised_Never_Events_policy_and_framework_FINAL.pdf.
5. Weich, B. (2016, January 27). 'Systemic failures' of NHS trusts led to the death of vulnerable 20-year-old Epsom mental health patient. *Surrey Comet*. Retrieved from https://www.surreycomet.co.uk/news/epsom /14225065.systemic-failures-of-nhs-trusts-led-to-death-of-vulnerable-20 -year-old-epsom-mental-health-patient/.
6. Provisional publication of never events reported as occurring 1 April 2021 – 28 February 2022.
7. Black, I., & Bowie, P. (2017). Patient safety in dentistry: Development of a candidate never event list for primary care. *British Dental Journal*, 222(10), 782–788.

8. Burnett, S., Norris, B., & Flin, R. (2012). Never events: The cultural and systems issues that cannot be addressed by individual action plans. *Clinical Risk*, 18(6), 213–216.

9. Burnett, S., Cooke, M. W., Deelchand, V., Franklin, B. D., Holmes, A., Moorthy, K., ... Vincent, C. (2011). *How safe are clinical systems? Primary research into the reliability of systems within seven NHS organisations.* The Health Foundation, 1–176.

10. BBC News. http://news.bbc.co.uk/1/hi/wales/2049839.stm.

11. Reason, J. (2000). Human error: Models and management. *British Medical Journal*, 320(7237), 768–770.

12. Queen's Printer of Acts of Parliament. (2009). The care quality commission (registration) regulations 2009. *CQC.UK*. Retrieved from https://www.legislation.gov.uk/uksi/2009/3112/contents/made.

13. Glasper, A. (2019). Implementing the NHS patient safety strategy. *British Journal of Nursing*, 28(15), 1030–1031.

30

Poor attitude

Health care professionals are expected to maintain a calm, collected and professional composure. Inevitably, though, there will be instances of dissatisfaction and complaints regarding the poor bedside behaviour of medical staff. Sadly, sometimes these complaints are justified. The pressures we face mean that we may be short with our patients at times. Recognising that and engaging coping strategies are important.

According to Gautham K. Suresh, disruptive behaviour is not at all rare in health systems.[1] At least 77% of medical personnel have confirmed seeing disruptive behaviour from physicians, and 65% reported to have seen it from nurses at least once in their career.[2] Usually, these are sporadic and do not represent a pattern of behaviour; however, they can be the source of complaints.

The poor attitude of doctors and health care professionals is typically the result of the high pressures inherent within modern health care systems. It is also true that often, the health care professional in question has more patients than they can handle or must work in situations they have not been trained for. Many doctors and nurses become embittered by the working conditions that they endure in health care, particularly in the NHS, with mounting pressures and tightening budgets.

The problem is compounded by the fact that throughout their training and careers, they may not have had any specific training on how to deal with confrontations and difficult pressurised situations. Often, they are thrown in the deep end and then face criticism when they sink and lose patience or their cool. Training for such circumstances is improving at medical school, but it is still not complete. According to experts, the cause behind rude behaviour is often 'physician burnout, poor stress management, poor self-care, and inability to manage the demands of work and personal life'.[1]

Despite a general understanding among the populace regarding the pressures health care professionals face, a patient may not want to understand or forgive the causes that lead a doctor to behave in an unfriendly manner. The best course of action is to recognise the nature of common complaints and grievance grounds regarding poor attitude and do our best to avoid incurring these issues by formulating coping strategies and enhancing training.

DOI: 10.1201/9781003179351-37

COMMON GRIEVANCES

The most common complaint of patients is that they do not feel heard. They often feel rushed and dismissed. For example, as quoted by Hogg et al., one patient complained, 'He (the doctor) did not give me any chance to put any of my points across or ask questions'. Another said the examination was rushed and she was told 'in an abrupt tone, not to be so stupid'.[3] Needless to say, these accusations can turn into formal complaints very easily, particularly if there is not a swift and satisfactory remedy.

If you find yourself in a situation where your patient is struggling to get their point across but you need to move on to another consultation, take some time to explain why you might not be able to give them the attention they want or need at that moment, but assure them that you will follow up with them later or that you have reviewed their tests thoroughly and are confident in the treatment. Usually, all patients need is assurance from their doctor.

When a patient comes to the hospital, they are there for a reason, so they expect the doctor to focus on that. Abrupt and unexplained changes in the treatment plan are also conceived as rude and belittling by many patients. For health care professionals, it is just another day at the hospital and another patient to treat, refer or discharge. For a patient, the experience is different. They expect their doctor to acknowledge their concerns about their health and behave accordingly. They expect time to put across their worries and a detailed and tailored explanation of their problem. If this expectation is not met, it creates a sense of less-than ideal service and lack of care/sincerity.

For example, a patient who has been referred by their GP for a colonoscopy may be unfit for the test due to obesity or may even not need the test because to an expert general surgeon, their diagnosis is clear.[1] Turning away the patient without any explanation regarding why they do not need the procedure or are unsuitable is undoubtedly unprofessional and will engender disgruntlement. Even if the patient is healthy, or simply needs antacids, their concerns are valid and need to be addressed. Failing to directly address them leaves the patient confused and feeling ignored and undervalued even though technically they were treated correctly in the medical sense.

A circumstance where the failure to meet expectations is likely to result in a complaint is when the patient is in pain. If a patient feels that they are being left to suffer and then, to compound it, the person they seek help from has a poor attitude and/or lacks sympathy, then they are more likely to complain, and often, this will be justified.

There is a significant psychological aspect to such complaints in relation to pain. For example, a pregnant patient admitted for delivery requires prompt care and pain relief. A study has shown that in up to 42% of cases, obstetric surgery had been allowed to start despite incomplete anaesthesia, and in 33% of cases, the patient actively asserted that she could still feel below her waist, but the anaesthetist rejected the idea that the nerve block was suboptimal.[4] In most obstetric claims regarding pain management cases, the doctor's (either the anaesthetist or surgeon) and nurse's/midwife's perceived unprofessional and unfeeling attitudes are the driving factors behind formal complaints and legal action.[5]

Hogg et al. reported that some complaints from patients recounted their experience as severely distressing, saying it left them 'angry', 'dejected', 'anxious', 'shocked', 'humiliated' and 'degraded.'[3] Their criticisms may be levelled at any member of the staff involved in the patient pathway. Feeling uncomfortable during testing, not being briefed before commencing with procedures or the staff being curt and unsympathetic to the patient's pain can influence the negative experience. Not only can this be the trigger for a complaint but also, such an experience can be a major factor in a complaint regarding another issue that would have otherwise been easily remedied.

When patients attend a health care provider service, they are usually in an extremely vulnerable position. This may be physical, such as they have been involved in a car accident and are bleeding heavily or they have broken their leg and need it set, or emotional pain/anxiety. Most patients are not asking for much. They expect and hope for good communication skills, clear explanations and a reasonable amount of patience from their doctors. We are all in the caring profession, and a decent level of caring is what patients do and should expect.

Directly rude or hurtful comments are solid grounds for a complaint, although by themselves, they do not tend to result in litigation. Nonetheless, they can seriously harm the reputation of a clinician or the service as a whole or even result in action from the professional regulator.

Recently, there has been a concerted effort to acknowledge and collect information regarding patient harassment and discontent. This has fuelled the number of complaints and potential medicolegal claims.[6] It is clear that bullying, harassment and other forms of unprofessional behaviour can result in action, even if they do not cause physical harm.

Rude behaviour should be addressed and not tolerated; however, not all rude behaviour will result in a sanction, and often, an apology can remedy the situation.

When dealing with patients, we remain human and are not expected to be robots. We can get frustrated or angry, but we are professionals and should not retaliate against patients. Doctors who have had to deal with a patient or their family being difficult and rude may feel that it is justified to also be rude in response. This is not a justification, and we need to hold ourselves to a higher standard than that of the patient, as they are in a distressed and vulnerable position, and their outburst can be acceptable.

Abusive and threatening behaviour does not fall into this category, however. If the patient is threatening physical harm, being racist, homophobic, sexist or shouting profanities, then the medical professional has the right to not treat them. This should be done formally and documented correctly. Sanctions are possible once the proper processes are followed, such as removal of the patient from a GP practice's patient list. Such actions need to be done by the book and with care, as the patient can raise concerns that they are being victimised or mistreated. The NHS has a zero-tolerance policy in effect that protects doctors and staff from violence.[7]

It is of note that unprofessional behaviour not only includes rude comments but also actions that do not reflect well on the profession. The Dr Simon Bramhall case is an example. Dr Bramhall was accused of branding his initials on the transplanted livers of the patients he operated on, without the patient's knowledge. He was accused and found guilty of assault by battery, although no actual bodily harm was done. The judge in charge of the case commented, 'This was conduct born of professional arrogance of such magnitude that it strayed into criminal behaviour'.[8]

This case is certainly unique but sets the rules for future cases with an understanding that any unexplained, indefensible behaviour on the doctor's part can be punishable by law if the court sees fit. Courts are not made up of fellow doctors but instead of lay persons who will not look kindly on the practices that may have been deemed acceptable and 'no harm done' in the past. The standards we need to adhere to are strict and enforceable. Furthermore, we owe it to the patients to make sure we live up to the trust they put in us.

HANDLING RUDE AND DIFFICULT PATIENTS

If a patient is rude or overly difficult, an appropriate course of action is to try and de-escalate the situation without having it result in a formal process. We can follow the DELUDE coping model,[9] which includes:

- Don't take it personally.
- Engage with the patient.
- Listen to the patient.
- Understand the problem and solution.
- Deal with it (compromise or say no if necessary).
- Escalate the concern (refer to a senior).

This may be easier said than done, and some patients will never be happy. Attempts must be made to resolve issues, as higher powers will not look kindly upon an apparent closed-door/freezing-out tactic to deal with a patient in distress, whether they are in the right or not.

GOOD MEDICAL PRACTICE

The GMC expects doctors to maintain a high standard, to be polite and considerate, to treat patients as individuals and with respect, to work with patients in a partnership approach and share all necessary information in detail, to advise patients and to support them.[10] At no point is a doctor allowed to discriminate, judge or attack a patient verbally or passively. All concerns and objections patients have should be treated with respect, and the patient should be made aware that they have the right to seek treatment elsewhere if they choose to. Maintaining these standards is not as difficult as it may seem.

Health care professionals and health care systems must actively work towards processes that reduce the chances of occasional negative behaviour by clinicians towards patients and to quickly and appropriately remedy any issues that occur. An overworked person is not a friendly one. Hospitals must increase their human resources so that doctors can work with patience without compromising on their professionalism.

The Hippocratic Oath states that a doctor will hold the needs of the patient above all other considerations. Doctors and the whole health care team need to recognise that the patient is the centre of everything they do and that an unhappy patient should be handled in a way that maintains professionalism and communication pathways.

REFERENCES

1. Gautham, K. S. (2020). Addressing disruptive and unprofessional physician behavior. *Joint Commission Journal on Quality and Patient Safety*, 46(2), 61–63.
2. Rosenstein, A. H., & O'Daniel, M. (2008). A survey of the impact of disruptive behaviors and communication defects on patient safety. *The Joint Commission Journal on Quality and Patient Safety*, 34(8), 464–471.
3. Hogg, R., Hanley, J., & Smith, P. (2018). Learning lessons from the analysis of patient complaints relating to staff attitudes, behaviour and communication, using the concept of emotional labour. *Journal of Clinical Nursing*, 27(5–6), e1004–e1012.
4. Mccombe, K., & Bogod, D. G. (2018). Learning from the law: A review of 21 years of litigation for pain during caesarean section. *Anaesthesia*, 73(2), 223–230.
5. Parliamentary and Health Service Ombudsman. (2012). *Listening and learning: The Ombudsman's review of complaint handling by the NHS in England 2011–2012*. Parliamentary and Health Service Ombudsman. Retrieved from https://www.ombudsman.org.uk/publications/listening-and-learning-ombudsmans-review-complaint-handling-nhs-england-2011-12.
6. National Guardian Freedom to Speak Up Office. (2020, January). *Speaking up in the NHS in England 2018/2019: A summary of speaking up to freedom to speak up guardians in NHS trusts and foundation trusts*. National Guardian Freedom to Speak Up Office. https://nationalguardian.org.uk/wp-content/uploads/2021/04/201920_ftsug_su_data_report.pdf.
7. Department of Health and Social Care. (2018). *Stronger protection from violence for NHS staff*. Department of Health and Social Care. Retrieved from https://www.gov.uk/government/news/stronger-protection-from-violence-for-nhs-staff.
8. "Liver branding" surgeon Simon Bramhall fined £10,000. (2018, January 12). *BBC News*. Retrieved from https://www.bbc.com/news/uk-england-birmingham-42663518.
9. Burnell, R. I. (2016). The right to be rude: Managing conflict. *Nursing Times*, 112(1–2), 16–19.
10. General Medical Council (Great Britain). (2024). *Good medical practice*. General Medical Council. Retrieved from https://www.gmc-uk.org/professional-standards/good-medical-practice-2024/get-to-know-good-medical-practice-2024.

31

Poor communication

The single biggest problem in communication is the illusion that it has taken place.

– **George Bernard Shaw**

Health care providers and patients have an interesting, complex and potentially fragile relationship. Historically, doctors are supposed to know everything, while their patients are expected to be uninformed and vulnerable. Whether treating patients or communicating with other doctors to find an ideal treatment plan, clear communication is always a must. Indeed, according to Huntington and Kuhn, miscommunication is the root of most clinical negligence claims.[1] This theory is confirmed by the findings of the 2015 CBS Benchmarking Report, which states that about 57% of malpractice lawsuits filed in the US were due to miscommunication between health care providers.[2] In the UK, the scenario is not significantly different.

According to the annual benchmarking report published by CRICO, 30% of all malpractice cases between 2009 to 2013 were due to miscommunication.[3] Alarmingly, the consequences of the communication failures were dire, as 44% of these cases resulted in severe patient injury, including death, and only around 7,000 cases incurred a total loss of US$1.7 billion.

According to the report of the PHSO in 2015, in almost all the litigation cases, a major contributor was communication failure 'between health professionals on the one hand and patients, clinicians and families on the other; clinicians and their teams; clinicians and other teams; and between hospitals and care providers in the community'.[4]

COMMON SCENARIOS RESULTING IN CLAIMS/ COMPLAINTS DUE TO MISCOMMUNICATION WITH THE PATIENT

A common cause for complaint is secondary to toxic/adverse effects of prescribed medications. Patients may have difficulty understanding the need for a medicine,

DOI: 10.1201/9781003179351-38

when and how many times they need to take it or which drug they should not take any more. For example, an older adult who was prescribed metformin is told that it will help him control his 'feeding urges', but he is not informed of his diabetes. So he stops taking the medication after a while, and as a result, his blood sugar increases significantly.

Explaining to the patient the importance and the function of the prescribed medicine gives them proper motivation to take it. The impact, although not always apparent, is statistically significant on the treatment outcome.[5]

Patients often complain about doctors who 'just don't seem to listen'. It is further compounded by the complaint that many patients feel as if their interactions with doctors are hurried. Doctors are, in fact, usually in a hurry. For example, in the GP world, with 7- or 8-minute appointment times and 30 patients to see, there is no alternative but to be in a hurry. The pressures of the system mean that we need to see high numbers of patients or operate on large volumes, and there is no extra time to spare with patients.

However, the way doctors communicate with patients has a great impact on the perceived quality of medical care, and often, the investment of a bit longer with a patient can prevent the risk of a complaint that will take several hours or even days to resolve. All health care professionals must ensure that the patient is listened to or, at the very least, feel that they are and that they are also listening.

Miscommunication can have serious consequences. This is highlighted by a case where a doctor failed to inform a patient of the common side effects of an anxiety medication he was prescribed. The patient subsequently drove after taking the drowsiness-inducing drug and caused a car accident, injuring himself and bystanders.[6] The doctor in this case would be found guilty if it is proven that the medication was the cause of the accident.[7]

If a delay in diagnosis occurs due to poor communication between the health care provider and the patient, an allegation may reveal that further injury resulted after treatment has been inappropriately delayed. It is often the case that a court will rule in favour of whomever they feel has suffered more harm as a result of another's actions – typically the claimant.

Doctors are also often reluctant to discuss end-of-life care because they fear an emotional response from their patients. However, poor communication in this critical phase of care has a deleterious effect on a patient's treatment decisions, symptom management, quality of life, expenses and mental health.[8]

Proper communication with the patient is also a key factor in avoiding litigation, even if there was a delayed or missed diagnosis. According to Schoenfeld et al., even if there is a missed diagnosis with an adverse outcome, patients are 80% less likely to pursue legal action against the doctor if they were part of the decision making.[9] A shared decision-making process, regardless of whether it is necessarily brief or thorough, assures the patient of their control over their own health and builds trust between the patient and physician. By contrast, being defensive or rude encourages distrust and subsequent litigation. A partnership approach is always key.

It is important for everyone involved in health care to understand that when things go wrong, patients want answers from their clinicians. Understandably, discussing mistakes or delays is difficult for both physicians and patients, but it is a critical juncture where common ground can be found. Handling it badly by belittling the patient or making them feel like they are not being taken seriously can polarise positions and make it impossible to de-escalate a situation.

It also helps to earn a patient's trust. A patient may be suffering from unusual symptoms that they will not mention if the doctor does not specifically enquire. The patient may also omit important lifestyle or medical history information. In fact, 26% of all patient–provider miscommunication relates to the patient's condition.[3] These often go unmemorised by the health care professional during a rushed clinic visit.

Building a bridge of communication with the patient encourages them to volunteer information they otherwise would not. Patients should do their part by being honest about their medical history but cannot be expected to do so. In turn, doctors have a responsibility to ask the right questions, and patients cannot be blamed for not volunteering pertinent information. If a patient is not clear about a symptom or any information, they can simply be asked 'can you please explain what you mean?' Asking questions builds understanding and trust. Documenting negatives to responses can be important too, as the assertion may be that the question was never asked.

INTERPROFESSIONAL AND INTERDISCIPLINARY MISCOMMUNICATION

According to the CRICO malpractice benchmark report in 2015, only 43% of incurred losses are due to patient–provider miscommunication, 73% are due to provider–provider communication failure, and in 16% of cases, they are due to both.[3] While the confusion or misunderstanding of a patient is understandable and even expected, from a health care provider, it will be considered a breach of duty.

A patient can be seen by a variety of health care professionals during their medical journey. This can result in conflicting opinions, misdiagnoses and mistakes. Patients often feel that they are being pushed 'from pillar to post' and never getting an answer. An area where we find ourselves at risk of complaint and litigation involves poor communication related to critical information exchange between doctors and nurses or other hospital staff members regarding inpatients.

A case report published by Manias et al. regarding clinical handover is an apt example of massive miscommunications.[10] According to the report, a patient was admitted to the emergency department of a teaching hospital for trauma from an assault to the face with a rock. When she arrived, the doctors stabilised her head and neck using a hard collar until spinal injury was ruled out, and her wound was left open for debridement. A CT scan was performed to fully assess the damage.

At the time of her admittance, one team had just finished their shift, and another was taking over. A multidisciplinary team, led by a senior consultant, handled the handover and gave verbal instructions regarding the patient's care. A number of clinicians were present, and the junior doctor who was in charge of the patient was standing at the edge of the cubicle. He did not hear the consultant's instructions to explore the wound and refer the patient to plastic surgery. Instead of asking to clarify the instructions, he read the medical notes and assumed the wound was explored.

Incidentally, the CT report was also lacking. It was never viewed in person; rather, a verbal report was received over the phone by the junior doctor, who then removed the collar, closed the wound with simple sutures and without any deep exploration, and discharged the patient. However, he did mention in the discharge paper that the GP should review the formal CT report and sent her a copy through fax, which was never received. He also had instructed the patient to visit the GP in 3 days.

The wound became infected within a few days, and the GP prescribed anti-biotics and analgesics to the patient. Two weeks after the initial incident, the senior doctor was made aware of the radiologist's report, which was amended the day after the discharge, adding that there was, in fact, a rock lodged beneath the patient's masseter muscle.

The patient was then recalled, but due to another team shift and miscommu-nications between the emergency department doctor and the plastics registrar, was sent home again. After another week, with help from the GP, she was able to receive surgery to remove the stone. By then, she had been unable to eat for weeks due to severe swelling of the cheek and floor of the mouth.

Thus, a gap in communication among the hospital staff is potentially disas-trous. Robust processes must be in place to ensure adequate communication, as well as safety nets to prevent communication errors/omissions resulting in avoid-able harm. Failing to communicate with members of the interdisciplinary team and between doctor and nurse or staff, pathologist and surgeon, or GP and spe-cialist consultants may lead to potential litigation if harm occurs. For instance, 43% of all anaesthetic injury-related claims involve *incomplete, inaccurate, absent or untimely* communication failures.[11]

Lack of communication between health care providers can lead to medication errors, unnecessary treatments and tests, delayed diagnoses and other problems that can be harmful to patients. Failure to communicate in a timely manner can also cause issues; for example, if a nurse caring for a patient overnight fails to alert the doctor to deteriorating observations.

STEPS TO TAKE

Eradicating hospital-wide miscommunication requires bold authority interven-tion. Having digital and backup data on all patients, meticulous record keeping and efficient, reliable and appropriate interpersonal communication building programmes and cross-training can prevent the worst mistakes.[12]

Medical professionals should take the initiative to be as specific and detailed as possible when orally or non-verbally passing information and instructions on to colleagues. The same attention to detail should be employed in recording patient details and interactions. Even among co-workers who have worked in a team for long periods already, keeping written records is wise. Also, establishing the practice of safety checks regarding critical clinical information among staff can be effective.[3]

REFERENCES

1. Huntington, B., & Kuhn, N. (2003, April). Communication gaffes: A root cause of malpractice claims. In *Baylor university medical center proceedings* (Vol. 16, No. 2, pp. 157–161). Taylor & Francis Group.
2. Hoffman, J. (2016). *Malpractice risks of healthcare communication failures*. https://www.rmf.harvard.edu/news-and-blog/newsletter-Home /news/2016/sps-the-malpractice-risks-of-health-care-communication -failures/.
3. Strategies, C. R. I. C. O. (2015). *Malpractice risks in communication failures*. Annual Benchmarking Report. The Risk Management Foundation of the Harvard Medical Institutions, Inc.
4. Parliamentary and Health Service Ombudsman. (2015). *Dying without dignity: Investigations by the parliamentary and health service ombudsman into complaints about end of life care*. https://www.ombudsman.org .uk/sites/default/files/Dying_without_dignity.pdf.
5. Kelley, J. M., Kraft-Todd, G., Schapira, L., Kossowsky, J., & Riess, H. (2014). The influence of the patient-clinician relationship on healthcare outcomes: A systematic review and meta-analysis of randomized con trolled trials. *PLOS ONE*, 9(4), e94207.
6. Edersheim, J. G., & Stern, T. A. (2009). Liability associated with prescribing medications. *Primary Care Companion to the Journal of Clinical Psychiatry*, 11(3), 115.
7. Florio, C. (2007). *450 Mass. 182; 877 NE 2d 567*. Supreme Judicial Court of Massachusetts.
8. Thorne, S. E., Bultz, B. D., & Baile, W. F. (2005). Is there a cost to poor communication in cancer care? A critical review of the literature. *Psycho-Oncology: Journal of the Psychological, Social and Behavioral Dimensions of Cancer*, 14(10), 875–884.
9. Schoenfeld, E. M., Mader, S., Houghton, C., Wenger, R., Probst, M. A., Schoenfeld, D. A., ... Mazor, K. M. (2019). The effect of shared decision-making on patients' likelihood of filing a complaint or lawsuit: A simulation study. *Annals of Emergency Medicine*, 74(1), 126–136.
10. Manias, E., Geddes, F., Watson, B., Jones, D., & Della, P. (2015). Communication failures during clinical handovers lead to a poor patient outcome: Lessons from a case report. *SAGE Open Medical Case Reports*, 3, 2050313X15584859.

11. Douglas, R. N., Stephens, L. S., Posner, K. L., Davies, J. M., Mincer, S. L., Burden, A. R., & Domino, K. B. (2021). Communication failures contributing to patient injury in anaesthesia malpractice claims. *British Journal of Anaesthesia*, 127(3), 470–478.
12. Foronda, C., MacWilliams, B., & McArthur, E. (2016). Interprofessional communication in healthcare: An integrative review. *Nurse Education in Practice*, 19, 36–40.

32

System errors

Anyone working within the NHS knows that the system is far from perfect. Each year, a high number of patients lose their lives or face permanent disability due to preventable mishaps. These system errors can be anything from user error or a software malfunction to poor design or inadequate training.

Continuous system errors are often due to institution-wide failures, such as problems with communication, system outages or poor record keeping through-out the medical process. Nevertheless, when we look at most clinical negligence claims as a whole, it is easy to see that many have nothing to do with technical abilities or clinical judgement. They have more to do with organisational failures, including processes and procedures that are poorly designed or implemented or both.

For example, about 237 million medication errors occur every year in England.[1] Errors in administration account for 54.4%, but 90% of them are harmless. The potential harmful errors, however, are prescription errors (33.9%), dispensing errors (17.5%) and monitoring errors (19.5%).[1]

Systematic errors in health care are typically the most difficult to prevent. Because they involve multiple factors and multiple people, it is unlikely that any one person can recognise the full scope of a problem and address it before it causes harm.

Moreover, system errors can occur frequently and go unnoticed due to their minor nature or the lack of direct harm they cause to the patient. These unnotice-able errors are known as latent failures because they lie dormant for some time before having an effect on the overall system, usually when they compound one another. After a time and in certain circumstances, latent failures become non-latent failures that can subsequently result in harm to patients.[2]

Not having standardised equipment is a common latent systemic failure.[3] If a hospital has several types of catheters, each type will require different connec-tions and setups. Yet not all frontline clinicians and nurses can be expected to be familiar with each setup. For instance, if a patient arrives in the emergency department who needs an intravenous catheter, the clinician may not be familiar with how to handle this particular catheter, and this unfamiliarity increases the

DOI: 10.1201/9781003179351-39

risk for an adverse event. This may be compounded by the use of locum doctors who are also unfamiliar with the equipment used in the hospital.

Another common yet preventable failure is the delay in referring patients between different departments of a hospital. These result in treatment being withheld unnecessarily for long periods and often worsening of the patient's condition. Delays to follow ups or failures to book follow-up appointments can also result in administrative breaches of duty due to system and process failures.

Some elements of system failure may contribute to clinical negligence claims or compound harm. These are often difficult to track and identify because they involve multiple points of failure within a complex network that spans several organisations and comprises numerous relationships between people, equipment, supplies and procedures.

For example, the lack of coordination between the staff, nurse and junior and senior doctors working on a patient is by far one of the most common system errors that leads to litigation. Systemic coordination failures, such as schedule conflicts and understaffing, lead to handover confusion, missing reports, mishandling files and repeating or skipping treatment steps.

Lack of staffing, poorly managed staff schedules that increase the risk of fatigue and error, poor infrastructure, unavailable or faulty electronic health records, unhealthy work environments, lack of standardisation of responses and blame cultures are often not recognised despite being the root causes.

In the Bawa-Garba case, for example, the junior doctor was made the scapegoat regardless of the obvious system failures. The trust investigating the case reported the systemic failures that were the major contributors to the patient's death, along with recommendations. However, this report was intentionally left out in the criminal trial, which declared Dr Bawa-Garba guilty of manslaughter.[4]

Later, the MPTS drew attention to the systemic failures again when they investigated the case fully and decided on a suspension of Dr Bawa-Garba.[5] They were serious enough that the Court of Appeal formally acknowledged these failures, stating them individually. The court also pointed out that the basis of GMC's appeal against Dr Bawa-Garba was to primarily 'maintain public confidence in the profession' and was not about whether the doctor was actually negligent.[4] The extent of the system failures was such that the Leicester Royal Infirmary staff had to take 70 individual actions to improve the condition of the paediatric ward.[5]

Such system failures as this are not rare, unfortunately. The Donna Ockenden report shook the nation with accounts of the failures of Shrewsbury and Telford NHS Trust. The report highlighted how, between 2000 and 2019, hundreds of babies died needlessly or suffered serious harm because of systemic failings and repeated mistakes. Ms Ockenden published two reports regarding this matter, one with 250 cases in 2017 and another larger review in 2020 with 1,486 cases.[6, 7]

The enquiry found 'deeply disturbing' failings at the trust where maternity staff lacked the proper training and skills to recognise the signs of danger in labour, fetal distress and maternal health decline. According to the report, among the 498 cases of stillbirth, at least one-fourth had major concerns about the care provided to the mother. In 29 cases, the babies lived to have brain injuries, and

65 developed cerebral palsy. The system failures that led to this massive tragedy were:

- A tendency of the neonatal department to not involve external specialists, such as paediatric surgeons and geneticists.

- Lack of proper protocols and significant delays: Patients were reported to be sent to the labour ward a good while after labour induction. Post-natal consultation was often delayed.

- Reluctance in proceeding to surgical management even when the condition of the mother clearly indicated a caesarean section: Even obstetric anaes-thetists were not called ahead, giving no chance of preparation for general anaesthesia. This closed and defensive culture was allowed to grow.

- Evidence showing that some of the staff were flippant and dismissive and had often used inappropriate language with mothers who were in pain or com-plained about the lack of quality care: Despite repetitive patterns of neonatal and maternal death, the system failed to make any changes.

- Staff shortages that led to some unavailable and overworked midwives who were not always able to provide the best care for the women and their babies; also, neglect was assumed to be the norm.

- Too many staff being inexperienced, while others lacked confidence to speak up if they had concerns; in addition, the staff members were untrained.

- Insufficient scrutiny of unusual deaths: The review team was told there was no recognised process or guidance for investigating cases where babies died unexpectedly in labour or within 7 days of birth.

- Pressure on families to not raise formal complaints and their concerns were met with derision and they were not listened to.

- Not following the national clinical guidelines: monitoring fetal and neonatal health was lax, and maternal health care was neglected, including mis-management of high blood pressure and gestational diabetes and failure to resuscitate.

- Failure to transfer patients to appropriate experts in time: actions were often taken too late, and the staff were not prepared to take timely action.

- Staff at the hospitals being bullied and intimidated into not reporting con-cerns they had regarding patient care.

Alarmingly, there was also a culture of mother blaming and undisclosed and undocumented facts regarding the conditions in which the babies died. On the rare occasions incidents were investigated, the methods were not up to standard. There was no accountability of senior staff or the hospital trust, and an environment of fear, denial and wilful blindness persisted.

The Paterson Inquiry showed similar situations in the hospitals Ian Paterson worked in. He was found to have conducted more than a thousand unnecessary surgeries that put his patients' health at risk. Reportedly, some patients were coerced, lied to and deceived into getting the procedure.[8] The hospitals and organisations who were aware of the situation failed to intervene or react. An utter failure of governance and a sheer lack of leadership, transparency and humanity were evident in both cases.

Without system reform, the quality of care cannot be elevated. The system failures have started conversations on how NHS trusts have been failing, especially in maternal and neonatal care, all over the nation.[9] Especially after the increasing concerns about the current system failures in health care, efforts have been taken to correct some of them. The formal recommendations in both of these reports include a multitude of actions.

The Paterson Inquiry, for example, pointed out how easily individual patient safety can slip through the gaps in the existing system. The recommendations include a single repository of all consultants, patient-involved treatment plans, transparency, standard protocols and the gap between responsibility and liability.[9] These regulations, when fulfilled, can moderate the actions of both private and government doctors and hospitals.

Almost all recommendations of these inquiries focus on reinforcing laws and upgrading the system. The system needs to incorporate a standard course of actions or protocols for all hospitals regarding patient complaints, recall patients, consenting procedures, patient rights, responses to unfavourable incidents (including proper investigations), the highest possible level of transparency, regulation and accountability. The correct approach to that goal is to focus on system conditions and appraisals and ensure the system is working for both doctors and patients.[10]

System conditions or factors, the lack of which leads to system errors, such as compliance with protocols or policies, availability of resources, patient load, staffing and supervision, are obviously not ideal in parts of the NHS. So, instead of individual staff-based practice, it is high time we focus on systems-based practice.

Systems-based practice is based on the understanding that many medical errors are caused by faulty systems, processes and conditions that increase the prevalence of people making mistakes or authorities failing to prevent them.[11] As we are coming out of the blame culture and into a healthier health care environment for staff and doctor alike, system reform is exactly what is needed to maintain quality.

This strategy for improving the quality of patient care focuses on the entire health care system, including the organisation and delivery of services and the environment in which care is delivered. This involves altering the system to be more patient-friendly and ensuring a healthy work environment. Patient safety can be improved by reducing human error and system fallouts, which can be achieved by increasing teamwork in health care settings, using evidence-based standards of care, ensuring the quality of each staff member and creating a learning- and transparency-driven environment.[12]

The renewed efforts to increase appraisal and revalidation seen in the NHS are certainly a step towards system reformation. Even though the focus is on the system, the individuals who work in the system must also ensure that they are capable.

Appraisal is a process through which a doctor's performance and achievements are assessed against the professional standards set by the GMC, along with locally agreed objectives. Revalidation is the process of periodic assessment to confirm that a doctor's knowledge is up to date and they are fit to practise in the UK. The GMC states that appraisals must be conducted at least annually and include certain topics, namely continuing professional development, quality improvement activity, significant events, feedback from patients and colleagues, and complaints and compliments.[13] These annual appraisals are necessary and timely given the current public opinion and need of accountability.

Additional efforts to increase the quality of care are also being undertaken. The government is to create a public repository with key information, to increase accountability in the private sector.[14]

Recently, the NHS has planned to increase digital involvement in health care by launching a federated data platform.[15] System failure complications, such as lack of coordination, delay in treatment and referral, and mismatching patient data or test history, can be expected to decrease if the whole system is digitalised. Doctors will still need to keep personal records and notes, but the blaming of individual personnel when the system fails will certainly decrease.

Reflecting on the Paterson and Ockenden incidents and other recent case law/reports, better teamwork, improved work environments and a culture of organisational accountability are needed. Programmes to increase teamwork, for example, can prevent most fatal delays and mistakes. Investment in staff and resources is also key to improve systems and protect patients.

REFERENCES

1. Elliott, R., Camacho, E., Campbell, F., Jankovic, D., St James, M. M., Kaltenthaler, E., ... Faria, R. (2018). *Prevalence and economic burden of medication errors in the NHS in England: Rapid evidence synthesis and economic analysis of the prevalence and burden of medication error in the UK.* https://www.bpsassessment.com/wp-content/uploads/2020/06/1.-Prevalence-and-economic-burden-of-medication-errors-in-the-NHS-in-England-1.pdf.
2. Lawton, R., Carruthers, S., Gardner, P., Wright, J., & McEachan, R. R. (2012). Identifying the latent failures underpinning medication administration errors: An exploratory study. *Health Services Research*, 47(4), 1437–1459.

3. Judgement of 13th August 2018, Bawa-Garba, C1/2018/0356, [2018] EWCA Civ 1879, paragraph 74.
4. Vaughan, J. (2018). *The long road to justice for Hadiza Bawa-Garba.* BMJ 2018;362:k3510.
5. Rodziewicz, T. L., Houseman, B., & Hipskind, J. E. (2021). *Medical Error Reduction and Prevention.* [Updated 2023 May 2]. In: StatPearls [Internet]. Treasure Island (FL): StatPearls Publishing; 2024 Jan-. Available from: https://www.ncbi.nlm.nih.gov/books/NBK499956/
6. Ockenden Review: Summary of Findings, Conclusions and Essential Actions. (2022, March 29). *GOV.UK.* Retrieved from https://www.gov.uk/government/publications/final-report-of-the-ockenden-review/ockenden-review-summary-of-findings-conclusions-and-essential-actions.
7. *Gov.uk.* (2020, December). Emerging findings and recommendations from the independent review of maternity services at the Shrewsbury and Telford hospital NHS trust. Ockenden Report.
8. Government Response to the Independent Inquiry Report into the Issues Raised by Former Surgeon Ian Paterson. (2021, December 17). *GOV.UK.* Retrieved from https://www.gov.uk/government/publications/government-response-to-the-independent-inquiry-report-into-the-issues-raised-by-former-surgeon-ian-paterson/government-response-to-the-independent-inquiry-report-into-the-issues-raised-by-former-surgeon-ian-paterson.
9. Dyer, C. (2022). Failure to work collaboratively and learn from incidents led to deaths of babies and mothers at Shrewsbury and Telford Trust, review finds. *British Medical Journal,* 376, o858. doi: 10.1136/bmj.o858
10. Bindels, E., Boerebach, B., Scheepers, R., Nooteboom, A., Scherpbier, A., Heeneman, S., & Lombarts, K. (2021). Designing a system for performance appraisal: Balancing physicians' accountability and professional development. *BMC Health Services Research,* 21(1), 1–12.
11. Johnson, J. K., Miller, S. H., & Horowitz, S. D. (2008). *Systems-based practice: Improving the safety and quality of patient care by recognizing and improving the systems in which we work. Advances in patient safety: New directions and alternative approaches (Vol. 2: Culture and Redesign).*
12. Carayon, P., & Wood, K. E. (2009). Patient safety. in K. Henriksen, J. B. Battles, M. A. Keyes, et al., editors *Information Knowledge Systems Management.* Rockville (MD): Agency for Healthcare Research and Quality (US). 8(1–4), 23–46.
13. General Medical Council. (2018). *Guidance on supporting information for appraisal and revalidation.* General Medical Council. https://www.gmc-uk.org/registration-and-licensing/managing-your-registration/revalidation/guidance-on-supporting-information-for-appraisal-and-revalidation
14. Mahase, E. (2021). Government commits to public repository of consultant details 'in principle'. *British Medical Journal (Online),* 375, n3115.
15. NHS England Plans Federated Data Platform. (2022, April). *UKAuthority.* Retrieved from https://www.ukauthority.com/articles/nhs-england-plans-federated-data-platform/.

SECTION 8

Speciality-specific litigation

Complaints, litigation, clinical errors are a part of life that cannot be avoided. Although we in the medical sector strive to be perfect at all times, it is impossible. The rush and the split-second decisions we need to make in the hospital or private practice mean mistakes will be made, and they sometimes lead to harm and potential litigation. Due to advances in science, complexities are increasing and making life harder for us all.

Sometimes, litigation occurs after small, trivial and negligible details that are easy to miss if we do not actively pay attention to them. Often, these are part of a chain of events where minor errors are compounded and escalate harm. Other times, the litigation is about serious issues that any doctor would want to avoid. With retrospect, these are usually obvious, and we are all at risk of succumbing to them.

The truth is mistakes are accidents, and there is never any malicious intent or volition. It is best to be aware of the common pitfalls, conditions, mistakes and technicalities that lead to litigation in our specialities so that we know how to avoid them. This cannot be an exhaustive list but simply a hint of the nuances of a specific speciality.

TYPES OF ERRORS: DO THEY VARY FROM SPECIALITY TO SPECIALITY?

Treating patients can be a repetitive experience, with diagnosis, advising tests and prescribing medications, and it is easy to make mistakes. Most patients' management is routine and will follow a well-trodden path. Each speciality is unique; however, there are certain patterns present in all. While these patterns assist in delivering standard treatment to all, they also mean that some mistakes are common. In this section, we will talk about the most common errors, claims and complaints of most specialities and how to avoid them.

DOI: 10.1201/9781003179351-40

33

Specialities

ANAESTHETICS

Researchers from the Association of Anaesthetists and NHS Resolution have published an insightful review of medical negligence claims related to anaesthesia. The review analysed all of the 1,230 anaesthetic negligence claims that were reported to the NHS Resolution between 2008 and 2018 and compared them to a similar analysis of claims from 1995 to 2007.[1]

Anaesthetists care for patients during approximately 4 million procedures in the UK or 3.3 million in England each year. In two-thirds of all admissions to hospital, an anaesthetist is involved in the patient's care. Despite the high volume of anaesthetic care, claims relating to anaesthesia represent only a small number and cost of claims arising from NHS care. Anaesthetic negligence claims increased by 62% in volume and by more than 300% in cost from 2008 to 2018, compared with claims from 1995 to 2007.[1] But those claims were only 1.5% of all claims submitted to the NHS Resolution and 0.7% of the total medical negligence claims costs, which were both lower than in the previous 12 years.[2]

The themes of successful claims resulting in settlements for the injured patient often involved:

- Inadequate anaesthesia (82%)
- Drug error (79%)
- Poor planning (78%), such as failure to recognise the higher risk status of patients with pre-existing health conditions (comorbidity)

The total costs (compensation and legal fees) were highest in anaesthesia-related claims involving cardiac arrest (£21 million), regional anaesthesia (£14.1 million) and drug error (£14.4 million). Two such claims arose from 'wrong route' drug errors involving the intravenous administration of large volumes of local anaesthetic, both with a moderately severe outcome.[2]

Obstetric anaesthesia

More than 75% of all anaesthetic negligence claims related to central neuraxial blockade, including spinal and epidural anaesthesia.[3]

Anaesthetic risk factors, such as maternal age and comorbidity, have increased over time, increasing the likelihood of complications. Despite its complexity and known risk profile, obstetric anaesthesia is more often classed as emergency work delivered by on-call staff and is commonly delivered by junior doctors without direct senior supervision.

A high proportion of claims related to pain or awareness during caesarean section and failed or repeated attempts at central neuraxial blockade (spinal or epidural anaesthesia).[3]

Airway management

Airway management is one of the most important facets of anaesthetics. Claims arising from negligent care of the patient's airway were infrequent (9%) but costly and, unsurprisingly, resulted in some of the worst harm, with 58% of patients suffering severe outcomes, including permanent neurological, respiratory and/or psychological injury. Almost one-third of all airway management negligence claims involved the patient's death.[4]

Central venous catheters

The safe management of central lines is the subject of numerous guidelines and standard operating procedures. Despite this, central lines are associated with claims for severe injury secondary to issues such as air embolism, infection, perforation, blockage or thrombosis. Only 2% of claims are related to central venous catheters, but the severity of injury – including 8% of deaths – and the average cost of these claims are significant and usually avoidable.

Cardiac arrest

Claims related to cardiac arrest are infrequent, with 1 claim per 50,000 anaesthetics, but the review emphasised that these are serious and very costly, averaging £631,000 per claim.

A quarter arose from drug errors, such as unflushed cannulae, wrong drug or incorrect drug dosage. One-fifth arose from errors in regional anaesthesia, such as epidurals and spinals. Fifteen per cent arose from airway management issues, such as an unanticipated difficult airway, problems with extubation and compromised post-operative airways.

Cardiac arrest was often the endpoint for the patient in the most significant adverse event claims. A quarter of anaesthetic claims arising from cardiac arrest were associated with death, but almost two-thirds involved severe outcomes. The high cost of these compensation claims was thought to arise from cases involving hypoxic brain damage and the consequent high costs of post-harm care needed for these patients.

Inadequate anaesthesia and awareness claims

A significant number of claims related to inadequate anaesthesia during monitored anaesthesia care, when residual muscle relaxant drugs were accidentally given through a cannula that had not been properly flushed, causing 'brief awake paralysis'. This can result in a highly unpleasant experience for the patient. This is hard to defend and is likely to lead to a significant compensation payout for significant psychological distress.

It is vital that drugs are labelled and colour coded and that cannulae are appropriately flushed.

Lack of informed consent

In all branches of medicine, informed consent is an essential part of the care we deliver. Failure to obtain the patient's informed consent was often a feature of claims relating to patients with severe outcomes. Sixty-two per cent of these claims related to permanent neurological injury from regional anaesthesia.[5] Whether the procedure was carried out negligently or not, the failure of informed consent breaches the duty of care to the patient. In many cases, the patient had not been given an explanation of alternative treatment options to the one provided.

Informed consent should be obtained and documented for all anaesthetic interventions. Furthermore, anaesthetists are expected to advise the patient of alternative forms of anaesthesia and pain relief. Discussion will be required with the surgical team, and it should be clear who is consenting to the patient regarding potential regional anaesthetic complications.

Monitoring failure/delay

Anaesthesia is an observation-driven speciality relying on active monitoring of the patient. Monitoring negligence claims included failing to identify adverse events promptly owing to poor monitoring or incorrect interpretation of monitors. Such failure to detect issues promptly results in delay and potential harm. The most obvious issue is a failure to note or respond to low blood pressure, resulting in neurological injury or cardiac arrest.

Anaesthetists must pre-empt and expect foreseeable complications and document them. Often, allegations about failing to consider potential issues can be easily defended by simply pointing to a list of the potential problems within the clinical record, showing that the doctor had considered the patient as an individual and tailored the care to them.

Meticulous record keeping and attention to detail are vital. Most anaesthetic claims are filed months or even years after the incident. Failing to provide detailed records of the events to the court severely undervalues the clinician's credibility. Contemporary notes are important; however, the court accepts retrospective notes as long as they are accurate and written as close as possible to the time of the incident.

Notably, most of these biases/errors occur with competent, dedicated and knowledgeable anaesthetists. In many cases, the errors do not result from negligence or lack of experience but rather from subconscious thought processes. Usually, focus and a habit of double checking are all that are needed. Anaesthetics is at its most challenging when things go wrong; therefore, all cognitive tools need to be primed to make handling the emergency as easy as possible.

EMERGENCY MEDICINE

In terms of errors and litigation, emergency medicine may be the worst of all specialities. According to Jena et al., at least 75% of all emergency physicians have been or will be sued at one point in their career, making it one of the riskiest specialties.[6] The number of patients seen in EDs and the variety of potential conditions compound the difficulty faced. A single shift in the ED can bring hundreds of patients with high acuity needs, many of whom are critically ill or injured. On top of that, emergency physician decisions are hardly ever black or white due to patient conditions constantly fluctuating. Often, there is no full past history, and doctors are forced to make potentially dangerous decisions based on snapshots of the patient's condition. Patients may be unable to accurately describe their symptoms due to pain or distress, or they may be unconscious or mentally impaired when admitted to the ED (e.g. in cases of drug overdose or major trauma). This dangerous mix makes the ED the riskiest area in the hospital after the operating room and the delivery room for litigation.

Some patients attend the ED in an injured or critical state; thus, any mistakes made by the emergency doctor have a greater propensity to cause death or grave harm. To compound this, probably more than in any other speciality, the difference between the expert sitting in their study or the judge in court scrutinising the case and the clinician on the front line treating the case live is greatest. In the cold light of day, the management plan may be obvious, but ED doctors do not work in ideal environments, and errors are a significant occupational hazard.

Hence, strategies to avoid litigation are preferable to fighting it.

The vast array of conditions that may present to the ED make it difficult to generalise about the root causes of most litigation against emergency physicians, but a few causes stand out, such as:

- Unsurprisingly, the most common reasons for clinical negligence claims against an Emergency Practitioner (EP) are that the doctor failed to treat an emergency appropriately and failed to reach the correct diagnosis.[7, 8] This is true for both adult and paediatric patients. For example, myocardial infarctions can be mistaken for dyspepsia or mechanical chest pain, melanoma for regular skin tags and appendicitis for a gastric ulcer.

According to Wong et al., the root cause of a missed or wrong diagnosis can be summed up as:

- Ordering incorrect investigations or failure to investigate at all (58%)
- Inadequate medical history taking and lack of thorough examination and assessment (42%)
- Incorrect interpretation of results (37%)
- Failure to refer (33%)

- A common claim against EPs is associated with a perceived standard of care or performance failure. A common theme running through numerous complaints and litigation is that the patient acknowledges they were diagnosed but the doctor had failed to provide the proper timely care needed. Most patients attending the ED need immediate attention, which can be hard to give in an emergency room filled with patients. Half of the litigation complaints were related to the unnecessary pain, distress, anxiety and uncertainty a patient suffered while they waited for the doctor, and the other half concerned the patient's death due to the lack of timely intervention.

According to Nowak et al., 1,500 deaths each year in the US are caused by delayed diagnoses and inappropriate treatments of anaphylaxis cases alone.[9] All clinicians/health care professionals should know the dosage and routes of important drugs such as epinephrine. Any personnel handling intravenous drugs should know how to manage anaphylaxis.

- A third allegation frequently raised against ED doctors relates to inadequate documentation. Innumerable cases are lost due to the lack of written accounts specifying the steps taken by the physician attending the patient. In the ED, this is vital and should be detailed enough for a court to determine the thinking process behind the decisions made. Red flags should be excluded and documented to be excluded. Serious differential diagnosis should be considered, documented and excluded with reasons.

Wrong decisions and wrong diagnoses will happen but do not equate to negligence unless the actual diagnosis was not considered and was discarded out of hand. Evidence for the clinician discarding an important diagnosis out of hand is clearly demonstrated by its absence from the clinical record.

- Drug errors feature highly in claims against EPs. These errors are relatively straightforward to investigate, and the error is usually very clear. Although they are tragic, they are entirely avoidable. In the confusion of the ED, particularly when dealing with acute cases in resus, it is easy to mix up drugs that sound similar. Even if the name of the medicine is not mistaken, the dose can potentially result in under- or over-treatment or severe harm/injury.

The experience of the doctor has a lesser effect in avoiding malpractice than one would assume. According to Carlson et al., the reason some EPs have faced more malpractice claims than others is that they were simply treating more patients than others.

Mistakes tend to occur in the ED more often in the following situations:

- *The night shift*: Clinical errors leading to ligation happen most often during the night or evenings. Naturally, doctors and staff are tired, and there are fewer staff on hand, less senior supervision and many unavailable facilities, such as CT and MRI.

- *Delays*: Waits are an inevitable part of a visit to the ED; however, a prolonged wait can cause anger and a sense of lack of care/neglect among the patients. This frustration pre-sensitises patients, and they are less forgiving of errors/issues than usual.

- *Shift changes*: These are typically staggered for doctors, but the change of staff can be en masse with the nursing staff. As a new team takes over, there can be a lack of continuity. Presumed differential diagnoses can become firm ones, while planned investigations can be overlooked.

    Communication and documentation are vital. If care is to be handed over, then a written plan should be in the clinical record. Ultimately, the blame is likely to rest with the clinician who saw the patient last.

- *Lack of informed consent*: This is always an issue that can result in litigation. This type of situation has become more common since the Montgomery case and the updated GMC guidelines.

GENERAL PRACTICE

General practice is the backbone of the NHS, and GPs see a huge number of patients. GPs are also the ones who must handle the widest variability in the nature and complexity of patients they see. They are the gatekeepers, the front-line triage clinicians and the ones at the coalface when it comes to spotting red flags and picking up the numerous masquerade syndromes/unusual/atypical presentations that others only read about in textbooks or case reports.

Conditions can range from minor to severe in terms of difficulty of diagnosis or rarity. General practice is a busy and complex environment, with consultations sometimes fragmented into brief appointments with several doctors, nurses or other health care professionals.

With the pressure of conflicting demands, it is not surprising that errors occur. This can be compounded by communication problems with other members of the team and between primary and secondary care. It is also important to recognise that at times, a patient's condition may be complex and difficult to diagnose and GPs are not expected to practice at the level of Dr House. The correct diagnosis may not be made at the first consultation even if all appropriate investigations are carried out. Getting a diagnosis wrong does not equate to negligence, but the patient is owed a duty of care, and the GP's conduct should be supported by a reasonable medical opinion.

A large number of errors in general practice resulting in litigation are not due to missed diagnoses but rather delays.

Most complaints feature some element of perceived or real communication failure. A patient may be unhappy because they feel that the GP did not listen to their concerns, failed to understand them or did not explain clearly what was wrong with them or what happened after referral to hospital. These complaints may be true or false, depending on what was actually said between the doctor and patient at the time of consultation.

According to several articles, delayed diagnosis is the most common allegation made against GPs.[10] In most courts, a GP will be judged against what would be expected from a reasonably competent practitioner, not the level of skill expected from a consultant physician or a super doc.

Avoiding litigation is probably impossible. The very nature of being a GP means that you will face patients presenting in a wide variety of ways. Mechanical-sounding chest pain may be the presenting feature of a myocardial infarction in otherwise healthy 40 year olds in 1 in 1,000,000 cases; however, that patient will walk through the door of someone's practice at some stage, leading to the incorrect diagnosis and maybe litigation. However, strategies can be adopted to try to reduce the number of claims made against GPs, such as:

- *Safety netting*: This was formally introduced nearly 30 years ago by Roger Neighbour,[7] who defined it as a process whereby the GP answers three questions: 'If I'm right, what do I expect to happen? How will I know if I am wrong? And what would I do then?' Safety netting is included in Neighbour's own model of the consultation, as well as the Calgary–Cambridge model, which includes safety netting in the section 'closing the session'.[8]

    > *Bankhead et al.[9] were among the first to attempt to provide recommendations for safety netting in primary care. They aimed to identify the components of safety netting related to cancer diagnosis and were the first to suggest that safety netting may be more than a consultation technique.*

    √ Clinicians should have documented a discussion with the patient on the problem of uncertainty, advice on potential red-flag symptoms, the likely time course of the illness, advice on the logistics and time for accessing further medical care, follow-up and the management of investigations. Safety netting may also include other factors, such as providing written information and documenting advice in the medical notes.
    √ Uncertainty exists in the majority of consultations, but without the first step of recognising and communicating uncertainty, the actual need for safety netting may be lost.
    √ It is important that patients do not slip through the net. Referral processes are not infallible, and the duty of care does not end once the patient has been referred to secondary care.

- Using the tools at the GP's disposal: GPs do not know everything about everything, but they can find out quickly. Generalist doctors are expected to know the basics of most specialities and how to conduct detailed searches for anything that they do not normally treat. The internet is an invaluable tool to assist in the work. The modern GP is familiar with a number of websites, and there are automated electronic assistance prompts in most Electric Patient Record (EPR) systems.

Colleagues are also an invaluable tool. It is important to ask if unsure or even if sure. In terms of litigation, the GP is effectively undertaking a mini-Bolam test if two GP colleagues agree with their diagnosis and management.

- Having a written complaints procedure that is available to patients: This procedure should explain to people how they can make a complaint, including who they should contact and what information they may need to put in. It should be published on the practice's website, which should be advertised within the practice. You are not afraid of complaints and want to learn from them to improve your care. You acknowledge as a practice that mistakes will happen and your duty is to reflect and learn from them. For example, the procedure may say 'if you have a suggestion or complaint about our practice, please let us know. We would welcome your suggestions about how we can improve the service that you receive from us'.

  After a complaint is submitted, it should be dealt with within 36 to 48 hours. If the complaint is in verbal form, a phone call should be enough. For written complaints, a formal apology or fix would be more appropriate.

- Keeping patient records: A well-kept record of patients is a legal requirement and also a valuable tool to avoid litigation. All records kept must be factual, concise and easy to read. The notes should be arranged in chronological order or in the order that consultations occurred rather than the order that entries were made. The individual patient record should also have sufficient detail so that another doctor or the court-appointed expert can understand the history, objective findings and grounds for any clinical management plan.

  In the era of EPRs, it is easy to use tick boxes, but a failure to tick a box may be seen as evidence that the question was not asked. Free text should be detailed so that a third party can understand the GP's thought processes. Differential diagnoses should be listed before picking the most likely one. For example, when facing a young patient with mechanical-sounding chest pain, the GP must ensure that it was stated that it did not sound cardiac. Failure to do so may mean that the GP failed to consider the most serious potential cause of the patient's pain.

- Not believing in self-labelled diagnoses: A patient may believe they have a chronic condition or have been diagnosed with one before. However, these are often misleading. This is an example of confirmation bias when clues are sought to confirm the diagnosis presented rather than trying to discredit it. For example, a patient may say they have a long history of sinusitis or tension headache when their pain is more in line with giant cell arteritis.

- Always checking for the one diagnosis whose miss cannot be afforded: No matter how unlikely it is, the worst-case scenarios should always be ruled out first and then be documented. Simple weakness and confusion can be dehydration or a stroke, and a blackening bruise in one's leg can be just a bruise or necrotising fasciitis. If a patient comes in with severe jaw pain, they should always be checked for angina or myocardial infarction. While it is unlikely, there is always a possibility.

- Failure to refer comes shortly after delayed diagnosis in terms of prevalence in letters of claim against GPs. If a GP fails to recognise that a patient needs to be referred to a specialist for tests or treatment, this can cause significant delays in the patient receiving the treatment they need. There may be pressure not to refer due to funding issues. Over-referral will be criticised as a poor use of resources, whereas under-referral can lead to disgruntled patients, harm, complaints and litigations. Administrative errors in relation to referrals, including patients getting lost in the system or a referral simply not being processed correctly by the GP surgery, can occur, so robust systems must be in place.

- Failure to follow-up or act upon test results: One of the hardest cases to defend is when an abnormal test result occurs but is not acted upon. The GP orders the test for a reason and is dutybound to act upon it. This can either be in the form of altered management or repeating the abnormal test. If the test result is clear and has been signed off by a GP, then it is clearly a breach of duty not to act upon it.

  In this situation, the following recommendations should be followed: Remedy the situation as soon as possible, be open and honest with the patient and make sure harm is minimised and assess the systems to determine how the error occurred and make changes to make sure the same thing does not happen again. Remember that harm has to occur to substantiate a valid claim. If no harm occurs, then a complaint may ensue, but litigation is unlikely to progress.

- Failure to act upon information: All health care professionals have a duty to care for patients and to act on information they receive from other health care professionals. If a GP, private doctor or hospital doctor receives information about a patient's health and fails to act in an appropriate manner and this failure causes the patient to suffer harm, then there may be an allegation of breach of duty.

  GPs face a vast volume of correspondence from other specialities and health care providers. Assessing and acting upon the appropriate parts of that communication can be hard, but processes need to be put in place to ensure that requests for further investigations or referral to other specialities are acted upon.

  With pressures in the health service and funding issues, patients are often referred back to their GP for referral to another speciality rather than an internal referral occurring. Even though the natural instinct is to think

> *'Why didn't they refer the patient themselves?' not acting or delaying can leave the GP open to criticism.*

- Communicating well: In specialities, communication is key. The doctor must talk to the patient and give them the time they need, if possible at their busy clinic. For patients who need it, a double appointment slot may be a sound investment of time. If disgruntlement is seen brewing, it should be nipped in the bud. The doctor should engage with the patient on matters of logistics and diagnostic uncertainties.

> *Doctors should acknowledge the pressures on the system. Patients do not expect them to be 100% correct all of the time. They are understanding of uncertainty and welcome engagement. Rather than saying 'it is definitely not cardiac chest pain', it is much more engaging to say 'I do not think it is cardiac chest pain because ... but if this occurs, then we need to think again'. If the pain is subsequently found to be cardiac, then there is no possible allegation of failure to consider.*

OBSTETRICS AND GYNAECOLOGY

Obstetrics is in the highest tier when it comes to litigation. Obstetrics is a field that leaves very little area for mistakes, considering the emotional and ethical responsibility, the delicate nature of the patients and the fact that the doctor is often simultaneously caring for two or more patients, some of whom may be inaccessible in the womb and only monitorable at a distance.

Given the prevalence of complications, the high number of clinical negligence cases is not a surprise. According to the NHS Litigation Authority, which is now supplanted by the NHS Resolution, from 2000 to 2010, there were 5,087 maternity claims, which accounted for a total of £3.1 billion – almost half of all compensation payout volumes.

According to the NHS Resolution Annual report and 2019/2020 accounts, 7% of claims were from gynaecology, and 9% from obstetrics, with a value of around £2,300 million.[11] In 2020/2021, the scenario was similar. Hence, the importance of avoiding errors, complaints and litigation in this speciality can be understood easily and has been the focus of numerous reviews and enquiries.

According to Bolcato et al., the medicolegal claims in obstetrics can be divided into six categories.[12] These are:

- Birth
- Antenatal diagnosis
- Pregnancy and after-birth period
- Treatment of gynaecological diseases
- Voluntary interruption of pregnancy (VIP)
- Artificial fertilisation or intrauterine device (IUD) positioning

While gynaecological claims were fewer than obstetrics, they were not less serious. The most common were failure to diagnose or treat diseases, procedural mishaps and VIP.[13, 14] In 2020/2021, most cases were regarding procedural mishaps during the placement of vaginal mesh, which has now been stopped.

The burden of harm in obstetrics affects not only the expectant mother but also the newborn and the future family. Harm to a baby can result in massive future care bills. Obstetrics is a complex speciality involving cooperation between different professional groups, including midwives, obstetricians and paediatricians; the necessarily uncontrollable and rollercoaster of events involved in every birth; and the active involvement of the mother giving birth during treatment.

A German study looked at preventable adverse events in obstetrics. They found that 44% of cases involved peripartum therapy delay, 36% related to diagnostic error, 34% to inadequate maternal birth position issues, 33% to organisational errors, 18% to issues related to inadequate fetal monitoring and 2% to medication errors. A significant number of cases with multiple errors were identified.

The learning points are difficult to generalise, but the common themes include:

- Communication is vital among the multi-professional team and also with the patient. Obstetric physicians also have to handle communication with family members, who may be distraught fathers or anxious parents. The delivery room is a scary place for most women, and when things are not going to plan, the tension can be extremely high. The patient not understanding what procedure is being performed on her or the doctor refusing to answer a patient's questions only adds to that stress, and some women may develop post-traumatic stress disorder, which obviously is a legal concern as well.

Good communication and rapport with the mother and father are important.

Patients are more likely to complain when they feel they have been misled or have not been made aware of their options before a procedure. A consistent approach with all patients concerning informed consent, including counselling patients about the risks, benefits, alternatives and side effects of all procedures and treatments, is standard. Consent in emergency situations from a mother who is already cognitively impaired by prolonged labour, pain, anxiety and/or blood loss is undoubtedly difficult.

- The most common allegations of negligence against obstetricians assert that a patient was injured as a result of negligent management of labour. Most complaints related to vaginal delivery and caesarean sections and the events occurring during delivery. Often, junior clinicians are managing these patients on the front line, and their lack of experience can be an issue.

- Detailed records and documenting all aspects of patient care are required for all patients, whether or not a complication occurs.

- The days when juniors used to pride themselves on never calling the consultant in should be long gone. The safety of the patient is paramount, and juniors should have a low threshold for calling in a senior consultant when complications arise, even if they feel confident they can handle it. Patient with placenta previa, abruptio placentae, previous caesarean section haemorrhage or pre eclampsia are at high risk of developing complications.

- Injuries to the newborn, including those resulting in brachial plexus palsy and cerebral palsy, are reasonably common. Some reasons behind the development of these palsies include failure to recognise developing or pre-existing risk factors, failure to perform shoulder dystocia avoidance manoeuvres and failure to assess the condition of the fetus and perform a caesarean section are common allegations.

- Uterine rupture is also a serious complication of vaginal delivery. This is especially a concern when the patient has had previous caesarean sections or has a uterine scar. Such patients should be appropriately consented and handled with care.

- An issue that can undermine a defence of negligence is the failure to assign the correct obstetric terms, such as 'failure to progress', 'prolonged second stage' and 'cephalopelvic disproportion'. If the defendant cannot provide the parameters of the exact conditions of the patient during the stages of delivery, it gives the court a sense of incompetence and disorganisation.

  Information regarding any prior delivery by the patient (how many and which type), the pelvic architecture, normal or abnormal fetal position, cranial shape, result of the Muller–Hillis manoeuvre assessment and the time and strength of uterine contractility should also be included in the clinical record.[12]

- Several cases related to screening tests, both invasive and non-invasive. For example, a patient saying no to an invasive screening test or saying they are unsure about an invasive test may not understand the conditions it screens. This patient may file a complaint later if her baby is born with Down syndrome. Patients choosing home delivery, or caesarean section or normal delivery should be informed about the risks and benefits of these options. All material risks should be explained in detail without being overbearing.

- The use of oxytocin for induction of labour is one of the most common interventions in obstetrics. Although this drug has a long history of safe and effective use, it comes with the risk of hyperstimulation, leading to fetal distress and caesarean delivery. To avoid complications, it is best to have guidelines in place on how much oxytocin can be used. In general, if oxytocin is given to induce, the drug should work on the patient within three to four hours of infusion. If the intended result is not achieved within this time, it is unwise to give more.

Full assessment and advice regarding the ways to avoid error and harm in obstetrics is beyond the remit of this text. The Healthcare Safety Investigation Branch's (HSIB) Maternity Investigations Programme and the Perinatal Mortality Review Tool (PMRT) were established in 2018. The remit of the HSIB maternity programme is to investigate a defined cohort of maternal and perinatal deaths and intrapartum brain injuries in babies. The remit of the PMRT is to review all perinatal deaths (i.e. stillbirths and neonatal deaths). The objectives of both programmes are to seek to identify the causes of these outcomes, including any underpinning systemic issues, in order to provide answers to families and to share any learning to improve safe outcomes in maternity and neonatal services. The outcomes should guide future attempts to avoid harm, which will then reduce the litigation burden.

ORTHOPAEDICS

With an ageing population, there is an increasing demand for orthopaedic surgery. This increase in demand has been accompanied by an increase in litigation and compensation claims.

In 2020/2021, there were 10,816 clinical negligence claims. Among them, 12% were against orthopaedic surgeons, making orthopaedics the speciality with the highest number of claims besides emergency medicine. In addition, orthopaedic injuries accounted for the highest number of non-clinical claims. Orthopaedic non-clinical claims were about 59% of the total claims. The value of clinical claims, by contrast, was only 3% of the total value, which was much less than from other specialities.

Lawsuits involving orthopaedic surgeons often centre on disfigurement, pain and loss of function because their work involves bony anatomy and muscular attachments. Often, orthopaedic issues can have a massive impact on the patient's quality of life. For example, an orthopaedic surgeon may have to tell a patient they can never play sports again because of an injury or they need to have their knee replaced. Unfortunately, it is easy for patients to direct their sense of hopelessness and anger after hearing this news towards the doctor caring for them. With the massive availability and prevalence of no-win no-fee solicitors, such patients can often seek to blame the doctor and commence proceedings.

Non-technical errors and litigation should be relatively easy to avoid by using the appropriate checklists, as suggested by the WHO, before, during and after surgery.[15]

As with all specialities, informed consent is always a major ground for potential litigation when there are surgical complications. Infection is another major complaint. Infection is a recognised complication of orthopaedic surgery, but claims can still succeed if a breach of duty/negligence can be demonstrated. Even if infection is on the consent form, it should be remembered that patients cannot consent to negligent treatment.

A French study retrospectively assessed clinical negligence claims and found that damages were sought for medical errors or treatment-related risk in 67.5% of cases and for failure to inform in 15.8%.[15] There was a suspected surgical site infection in 79.3% of cases, and there were multiple grounds for complaint in 68.3% of cases. Poor communication between the physician and patient was identified in 26.2% of cases.

Harm includes further damage sustained unintentionally while preparing the patient, dropping the patient, failure to provide the best care post-operation, failure to adhere to local protocols, failure to refer, presence of chronic pain after surgery and choosing the wrong implant size, and these are all examples of successful claims against orthopaedic surgeons.

Measures to avoid complaints, harm and litigation in orthopaedics are similar to those for other specialities, such as:

- Use methodical history taking, examination and investigation to arrive at a diagnosis. The full range of diagnoses, including all differential diagnoses, must be considered and documented. Following local or published guidelines in treating difficult cases ensures the doctor is safe, regardless of the outcome. Most courts will ask for the opinion of an expert, who in turn will judge the action of the defendant based on standard practice guidelines. Usually, errors do not adversely affect the outcome.

  > For example, Gidwani et al. described two cases admitted with post-trauma fractures. One had a significant delay in diagnosis and treatment, while the other had a lack of informed consent. When brought before the court, the consensus expert opinion was that the outcomes of both cases were not affected by the breaches of duty. Hence, despite the presence of breach of duty, the cases were dropped.[16]

- Always record the findings in writing and make sure they are clear and legible. Documentation is what saves or condemns the surgeon. Courts place much emphasis on contemporaneous notes.

- Avoid long delays in operating on fractures and dislocations unless clinically justifiable. Patients want their remedial surgery as quickly as possible, and they may blame any poor outcome on the delay to surgery.

- In cases of chronic pain or disability, the patient should receive appropriate physiotherapy and other non-surgical management before the operation. Document that alternative treatments were discussed.

- In case of complicated surgeries, a consultant should at least be present, if not performing the surgery themselves.

- If something goes wrong, inform the patient immediately after surgery in a calm manner. The duty of candour must be fulfilled, and the patient must be fully informed of the complication and the possible detrimental sequelae.

- Mistakes such as skin burns, tourniquet injuries and medication errors can be avoided with appropriate care. Such errors are usually indefensible, and the entire team is responsible for ensuring they do not occur.

- Seek a second opinion if the patient's expectations or demands are difficult to meet and you are not sure of the successful outcome. It is better to refer the patient to a colleague who did not have surgery rather than one who already had an unsuccessful or unnecessary one. Unfortunately, the 'I told you so' defence may not be successful, as we are duty-bound not to inflict unnecessary harm.

- Good post-operative care is vital in reducing litigation. Good liaison with the recovery staff, ward staff, on-call team and anaesthetist is important. Ensure that the patient is getting their antibiotics, venous thromboembolism prophylaxis, physiotherapy, regular dressings and appropriate fluids.

- Arthroplasty surgeons see a high proportion of claims because of failure to diagnose neurological deficits and infection.[17, 18]

- Wrong-site surgery still occurs. It is entirely avoidable, and pathways should be in place to make sure it never happens.

- It is important that all imaging is available for clinic attendances or operative procedures.

The consultant orthopaedic surgeon is the team leader as captain of the ship and is held accountable for clinical errors. Skevington et al. described the environmental, systematic, psychological and organisational factors that contribute to consultant surgeons making avoidable errors.[17] Such factors must be recognised and reflected upon to avoid errors in the future.

Check listing the surgical procedure in the perioperative period is essential and requires a team-based approach. It should not be a simple tick-box exercise.

RADIOLOGY

Radiology claims are reasonably low, considering how many cases are handled each day. However, when considered as part of the overall burden on health care resources, particularly in terms of litigation costs and clinical time, they remain an important consideration. Radiological reports are considered definite information regarding the patient and are rarely challenged. As clinicians across the UK depend on radiological findings for the diagnosis and treatment plan, misdiagnosis can have grave consequences for patients and for the people who care for them.

According to Hulson, the most common claims between 1995 and 2014 were based on missed diagnoses of tumours.[19] The reasons were mostly simple human error: missing or misinterpreting a tumour, fracture or other abnormality that should have been detected. Other causes included delays in reporting, which should be done within 24 hours, poor communication with referrers and lack of follow-up after an inconclusive scan or treatment plan that deviates from standard practice.

Radiologists are required to interpret thousands of images every day under pressure and tight deadlines. They are also expected to work in high-tech environments that increasingly use automated processes and algorithms to aid with diagnosis. Although the potential benefits offered by artificial intelligence are significant, there is still no substitute for experience, expertise and common sense when it comes to interpreting X-rays and scans.

Interventional radiology may seem like a high-risk area; however, claims are surprisingly low. When claims do occur, they typically involve post-procedure bleeding, substandard technique (almost 50%) and failure to obtain consent.

Compared to this, non-clinical departmental injuries are higher in number and much more likely to result in a claim. These are not related to the treatment of radiology at all but rather adverse accidents, such as falls. Examples of in-department injuries include having a patient in the MRI suite even though they have a permanent cardiac pacemaker, placing a heavy oxygen cylinder close to the private parts of a male patient, resulting in injury, and a patient sent to the MRI suite without removing their hearing aids and metal body accessories.[19]

According to Craciun et al., a few preventive measures can significantly reduce the risk in the radiology department.[20] They recommended the following:

- Quality assessing and enforcing systems, such as quality maps, measurable metrics and performance indicators for audit and accreditation programmes, should be in place. A beneficial practice is to follow the 'as low as reasonably practicable' routine, which entails assessing risks and comparing them to the resources needed to address them. The idea is that residual risk can be reduced as much as reasonably possible. Another way of saying this is that if there is a potential risk in the department, all attempts within reason should be made to avoid it.

- A *clear disclosure* after any radiological errors can help to avoid most radio-logical claims. The key is to catch the error as quickly as possible and to report it to the associate doctor or surgeon so that any potential delays can be mitigated.

- Being available for phone calls from clinicians and actively calling clinicians when there are doubts or concerns about an image can help both avoid litigation that stems from missing critical findings on an image.

- Being up to date in the latest technology and techniques is important. Failure to refer to regional centres if they have a more appropriate imaging device can result in a claim.

- Proper written information should be given in the form of leaflets and sheets. Also, all the information given to the patient and communications with clinicians and patients must be documented in the medical record to ensure the doctor's version of events is on record in case there is a later dispute about what information was or was not provided.

- Written consent should be required for unusual patients. This is especially important for patients who have a history of mental illness or substance abuse. If the patient has any history of violent or irrational behaviour, they should be required to sign paperwork that states they are aware of the risks of their treatment and agree to the terms.

Radiology is particularly vulnerable to framing bias in that the clinician can focus on the presumptive diagnosis and on that area on the imaging while missing some other lesion. A classical example is missing an anterior brain tumour when imaging is requested querying a cerebellar or brain stem issue.

REFERENCES

1. Oglesby, F. C., Ray, A. G., Shurlock, T., Mitra, T., & Cook, T. M. (2022). Litigation related to anaesthesia: Analysis of claims against the NHS in England 2008–2018 and comparison against previous claim patterns. *Anaesthesia*, 77(5), 527–537. doi: 10.1111/anae.15685

2. How common is anaesthetic negligence? NHS resolution and the association of Anaesthetists' review of claims related to anaesthesia (2022, March 9) *Boyes Turner*. Retrieved from https://www.boyesturnerclaims .com/news/how-common-anaesthetic-negligence-nhs-resolution-and -association-anaesthetists'-review-claims.

3. McCombe, K., & Bogod, D. G. (2018). Learning from the law: A review of 21 years of litigation for pain during caesarean section. *Anaesthesia*, 73(2), 223–230.

4. Singh, M., Liao, P., Kobah, S., Wijeysundera, D., Shapiro, C., & Chung, F. (2013). Proportion of surgical patients with undiagnosed obstructive sleep apnoea. *British Journal of Anaesthesia*, 110(4), 629–636. https://doi .org/10.1093/bja/aes465.

5. Pearson, A., & Cook, T. (2017). Litigation and complaints associated with day-case anaesthesia. *BJA Education*, 17(9), 289–294.

6. Jena, A. B., Seabury, S., Lakdawalla, D., & Chandra, A. (2011). Malpractice risk according to physician specialty. *New England Journal of Medicine*, 365(7), 629–636.

7. Wong, K. E., Parikh, P. D., Miller, K. C., & Zonfrillo, M. R. (2021). Emergency department and urgent care medical malpractice claims 2001–15. *Western Journal of Emergency Medicine*, 22(2), 333.

8. Selbst, S. M., Friedman, M. J., & Singh, S. B. (2005). Epidemiology and etiology of malpractice lawsuits involving children in US emergency departments and urgent care centers. *Pediatric Emergency Care*, 21(3), 165–169.

9. Nowak, R., Farrar, J. R., Brenner, B. E., Lewis, L., Silverman, R. A., Emerman, C., ... Wood, J. (2013). Customizing anaphylaxis guidelines for emergency medicine. *Journal of Emergency Medicine*, 45(2), 299–306.

10. Neighbour, R. (1987). *The inner consultation*. Radcliffe Publishing Ltd.

11. NHS Resolution annual reports and accounts 2019/20. https://resolution
    .nhs.uk/wp-content/uploads/2020/07/NHS-Resolution-2019_20-Annual
    -report-and-accounts-WEB.pdf
12. Cohen, W. R., & Schifrin, B. S. (2007). Medical negligence lawsuits relat-
    ing to labor and delivery. *Clinics in Perinatology*, 34(2), 345–360.
13. Bolcato, M., Fassina, G., Borgato, I., Sanavio, M., Rodriguez, D., & Aprile,
    A. (2020). Obstetrics-gynecology litigation 17 years of medico-legal
    experience in professional liability watchdog. *Acta Medica Mediterranea*,
    36(5), 3161–3166.
14. Hüner, B., Derksen, C., Schmiedhofer, M., Lippke, S., Janni, W., & Scholz,
    C. (2022). Preventable adverse events in obstetrics—systemic assess-
    ment of their incidence and linked risk factors. *Healthcare*, 10(1), 97.
15. Mouton, J., Gauthé, R., Ould-Slimane, M., Bertiaux, S., Putman, S., &
    Dujardin, F. (2018). Litigation in orthopedic surgery: What can we do to
    prevent it? Systematic analysis of 126 legal actions involving four uni-
    versity hospitals in France. *Orthopaedics & Traumatology: Surgery &
    Research*, 104, 5–9.
16. Gidwani, S., Zaidi, S. M. R., & Bircher, M. D. (2009). Medical negligence
    in orthopaedic surgery: A review of 130 consecutive medical negli-
    gence reports. *Journal of Bone and Joint Surgery, British Volume*, 91(2),
    151–156.
17. Skevington, S. M., Langdon, J. E., & Giddins, G. (2012) 'Skating on thin
    ice?' Consultant surgeon's contemporary experience of adverse surgical
    events. *Psychology, Health & Medicine*, 17, 1–16.
18. Bhutta, M. A., Arshad, M. S., Hassan, S., & Henderson, J. J. (2011). Trends
    in joint arthroplasty litigation over five years: The British experience.
    Annals of the Royal College of Surgeons of England, 93(6), 460–464.
19. Hulson, O. (2018). Litigation claims in relation to radiology: What can we
    learn?. *Clinical Radiology*, 73(10), 893–901.
20. Craciun, H., Mankad, K., & Lynch, J. (2015). Risk management in radiology
    departments. *World Journal of Radiology*, 7(6), 134.

SECTION **9**

Learning and avoiding errors

34

How we learn

As professionals in a field that is ever-changing, health care professionals are expected to keep their knowledge up to date and skills sharp. Moreover, while the curriculum of medical schools and nursing schools tries to be thorough, all health care professionals have to relearn and modify much of it when they start practising in the field and refresh their knowledge on a periodic basis as science and technology improve.

Junior doctors, especially, are often expected to memorise an immense amount of data and procedures in very little time as they train in every branch of health care. Often, they are thrown in the deep end and expected to know everything in a short period.

Guidelines change and evolve, and if we do not adhere to them, we can be criticised. If we allow our knowledge to become out of date, we can fall afoul of a clinical error that may be indefensible.

The GMC guidance on keeping up to date includes:

- Responsibility for identifying our needs and planning how to address them
- A requirement to reflect regularly on the standards of our medical practice
- Remaining competent and up to date across the scope of our medical role
- Maintenance and improvement of the standards of our practice and that of the team in which we work

Every health professional needs to learn throughout their career, so it is important to focus on how we learn and what learning techniques work for us. Care professionals have limited time and thus need to maximise learning efficiency.

According to Mayer, 'Learning is the relatively permanent change in a person's knowledge or behaviour due to experience'.[1] According to Wade et al., learning, or more precisely, memorising, is all about reciting what one has read or memorised. They support the 3R technique – read, recite, review – for optimal effective learning, especially for students.[2]

DOI: 10.1201/9781003179351-43

THEORIES OF LEARNING AND HOW THEY APPLY TO HEALTH CARE PROFESSIONALS

Learning theories are organised frameworks for understanding how individuals acquire and retain knowledge. They provide explanations for how we learn, including the thought processes that take place during learning events. There are a few theories on how professionals such as doctors and nurses learn at their job. According to Taylor and Hamdy, like most other individuals, the general theories of adult learning apply to health care professionals as well.[3]

INSTRUMENTAL LEARNING THEORIES

- **Behavioural theories**: People learn to change their behaviour following a stimulus in the environment. This is the most basic theory of learning that applies to the animal kingdom. For health care professionals, this theory applies when taking exams, followed by positive reinforcement of the desired results with grading systems.[4] In everyday hospital settings, this may translate to patients getting well or the rapport and respect a professional builds among their colleagues and seniors. The theory is applicable for continuous professional development.

- **Cognitive learning theories**: These are based on perception and the processing of information in the mind of the individual.[5] For health care professionals, this theory mostly applies to undergraduates. Cognitive learning applies to doctors and nurses when they apply the theories they learned to come up with new solutions or techniques to treat a patient.

- **Experiential learning**: Experiential learning theory 'focuses on developing competences and practising skills in a specific context'.[6] Simply put, experiential learning is the process of learning through experience. The most widely used model of experiential learning is Kolb's, who proposed that one learns from concrete experiences, which are transformed into reflective observations and then into abstract concepts (or observations), which are then used to create new experiences.[7]

The importance of experiential learning in medicine is obvious. We learn from our mistakes and successes, as well as from those of others. In the practice of medicine, we often rely on our own experience but have to be aware that this may not be enough. We have to augment it with guidelines and evidence-based protocols, both of which often come from places and times that may not be directly applicable to our situations. Nevertheless, it is important to encourage and practise experimentation or doing. For example, a nurse in training will remember the procedure to place an IV catheter for longer and more accurately when they practise it rather than just read about it.

HUMANISTIC THEORIES

Humanistic theories of learning are based on the premise that humans are active, not passive, participants in their own learning.[8] These theories are more individual centred. Although a doctor's journey begins with mastering the theory and practice of medicine, it continues with the development of their personal style as a physician. The same applies to all avenues of health care. Self-actualisation is attained through one's own knowledge and skills and the need to improve as an individual.

Knowles' theory of andragogy, or adult learning, is based on the following assumptions that fit health care professionals perfectly: they are self-directed, are problem centred, bring life experiences and knowledge to learning experiences, are goal oriented and are relevance oriented.[9] As health care professionals, self-improvement and self-directive methods of learning are apt when expected to direct and take responsibility as a senior.

TRANSFORMATIVE LEARNING THEORY

Transformative learning theory is about critical reflection on our beliefs and thoughts. This theory is based on the form of learning that involves significant changes to the way that we perceive our world.[10] In medical education, this can be practised when a critical or rare case is presented or through group discussions, idea presentations, etc. [11] This is a good exercise for junior medical professionals, as it teaches them to think elaborately and with an open mind.

According to this theory, people learn by experiencing a transformative crisis that challenges their assumptions. When faced with such a crisis, we must be able to confront these dilemmas. Through these methods, we can learn to let go of our previous presumptions and open up to new medical procedures and protocols. Specifically, having regular discussions regarding new developments teaches doctors not only about the medical inventions themselves but also how to broaden our minds and learn to learn.

SOCIAL THEORIES OF LEARNING

The social theories focus on context and community. Social learning theory is an approach to understanding the learning process. This theory, which draws on ideas from social psychology and developmental psychology, focuses on the importance of observing and modelling others' actions, beliefs and behaviours.[12] According to this theory, people learn not just by doing but also by observing others' actions and attitudes and the outcomes of those actions.

For example, health care professionals often perform procedures and duties in a specific manner, mirroring what they observed their teachers doing during training.[13]

The theory is partly true in medicine. Physicians often follow their mentors' methods and techniques. However, as a medical professional is expected to work with many teams, being flexible is more beneficial to the patient. Junior doctors or trainee professionals usually do things 'because that's the way it is done', but we should understand why certain things are done in specific ways before we choose to follow them. Evidence-based practice is key, and the health care field should avoid learning in silos. Modern technology allows knowledge sharing on an unprecedented level, and we should strive to use it to further learning and patient care.

MOTIVATIONAL MODELS

Motivational models are theories explaining the motivation and reflection behind learning. Self-determination theory, a popular motivational model, matches the motivation seen in medical training. The theory states that the factors working behind self-motivation are autonomy, competence and relatedness.[14] Students or health care professionals who feel that their place in medical society is earned or have a feeling of belonging are more likely to have a higher intrinsic motivation to learn. As they are entrusted with responsibilities, their faith in themselves increases, along with the feeling of belonging and competence, leading to higher motivation. Clearly, the trust and respect of our patients should be the driving force behind our need to keep up to date.

REFLECTIVE MODELS

Reflective models of learning emphasise learning from experiences. The reflection-change model hypothesises that reflection leads to action and then change. In this model, the health care professional's experiences lead them to reflect on their actions, consider alternative actions and make changes for the future. The advantage of this is that it gives practitioners a chance to develop their own insights into their work and apply them to future practice.[15]

Reflection-in-action and reflection-on-action are two types of reflective learning. Reflection-in-action suggests that thinking is an integral part of the situation, while reflection-on-action suggests that the thinking process happens after the situation has been experienced. Without doubt, both are invaluable in medical practice.

According to the GMC, all doctors should regularly reflect on their actions.[16] There is an emphasis on reflective learning, requiring health care professionals to submit written or verbal reflections of cases and what they learned from them during the appraisal process. We are bound to make mistakes. According to specialists, reflecting on these mistakes encourages medical professionals to be competent and acquire deeper clinical knowledge.[17]

CONSTRUCTIVISM

Like reflection, a cognitive constructive approach to learning is perhaps more suited to health care professionals than other methods. Constructivism focuses on 'the internal cognitive mechanisms that underlie the learning processes, participation, and social interaction' and is outcome based.[18] In the medical profession, this translates into strategies such as group discussions, journal clubs, critical appraisals and case presentations.

CONTINUOUS PROFESSIONAL DEVELOPMENT

Continuous professional development (CPD) is expected of all practising health care professionals, no matter where they are in their career. In other words, they are expected to learn in a continuous manner and keep updating their skills.

The GMC mandates training for all health care personnel as part of their appraisal process to keep up their personal CPD. Doctors are also required to keep a portfolio of evidence showing how they have fulfilled the requirements for revalidation.

The GMC requires all doctors to take part in, document and reflect on CPD activities. This is the first of the six types of supporting information a doctor must collect for their appraisal. While CPD activities and their impact are discussed with the appraiser, the GMC does not control which CPD method is chosen, as long as it is appropriate.[19]

The methods of CPD vary depending on the sub-speciality and individual choice. CPD activities can include:

- Work-based assessments
- Learning from experience, including reflective practice and supervision
- Learning from others, including mentoring and educational supervision
- Participating in research projects or audit projects
- Formal courses, such as conferences or courses run by approved organisations
- Work shadowing and secondments
- Professional reading of, for example, journals or books

According to Manley et al., based on the analysis of the outcome and the CPD methods, the effectiveness of a particular method depends on why it was employed.[20]

For example, a physician or practice having concerns regarding workplace efficiency or having available CPD opportunities will unconsciously seek out CPD focusing on workplace issues. Hence, the outcome of a CPD method for this particular team is likely to be improved efficiency and teamwork.

The nature of CPD also reflects the environment of the workplace. According to Manley et al., when the context is a workforce that is aware of the necessity of improving its skills, it creates a knowledge-rich environment and supportive workplace culture that draws out active contributions from the employees to practice development.[20]

BEST METHODS FOR LEARNING

One size does not fit all with regard to learning. While there is no exact method that works best, a combination of techniques to engage the whole team reduces mistakes and enhances safe and effective care. Cross-training or cross-learning is key for maintaining safety and improving service quality. If every individual in the team is involved in training initiatives, it allows them to work together smoothly, eliminating system failures.

For example, a nurse's primary focus is on patient care, not record keeping, but they fill in for a receptionist who regularly tracks patient appointments and phone calls and is also responsible for tracking incoming emergencies. Lack of coordination between them will eventually result in detriment to patients coming to the hospital who may have an undue wait before they are treated.

Additionally, an administrative professional may not have the same knowledge of patient care as a registered nurse, so even simple tasks such as scheduling follow-up appointments can become complex. Surgical teams also benefit from team-wide training. Alternatively, modular training techniques offer surgical teams learning opportunities better tailored to their needs.

For instance, a complex laparoscopic procedure, such as endoscopic extraperitoneal radical prostatectomy, is difficult to learn even when observing directly.

Dividing it into several levels or modules (12 individual steps, in this case) depending on their difficulty offers many advantages: it reduces the learning curve by several orders of magnitude, allows training at several sites, reduces exclusivity and allows even a beginner to train in a complex surgery.[21] The modular method of training can be applied to most other specialities if needed. Modern medical learning requires adaptability and short learning curves in order to be efficient.

REFERENCES

1. Adebiyi, A. (2019). *Understanding effective learning.* https://www.linkedin.com/pulse/understanding-effective-learning-adebayo-adebiyi.
2. Wade, C., Tavris, C., & Garry, M. (2014). The nine secrets of learning. *Psychology.* https://www.apa.org/ed/precollege/psn/2013/09/learning-secrets.
3. Taylor, D. C., & Hamdy, H. (2013). Adult learning theories: Implications for learning and teaching in medical education: AMEE guide no. 83. *Medical Teacher*, 35(11), e1561–e1572.
4. Kay, D., & Kibble, J. (2016). Learning theories 101: Application to everyday teaching and scholarship. *Advances in Physiology Education*, 40(1), 17–25.
5. Gagne, R. M., & Briggs, L. J. (1974). *Principles of instructional design.* Rinehart & Winston.
6. Yardley, S., Teunissen, P. W., & Dornan, T. (2012). Experiential learning: AMEE guide no. 63. *Medical Teacher*, 34(2), e102–e115.

7. Morris, T. H. (2020). Experiential learning–A systematic review and revision of Kolb's model. *Interactive Learning Environments*, 28(8), 1064–1077.
8. Rogers, C. R. (1963). Toward a science of the person. *Journal of Human Psychology*, 3, 72–92.
9. Knowles, M. S., Holton, E. F. III, & Swanson, R. A. (2014). *The adult learner: The definitive classic in adult education and human resource development*. Routledge.
10. Mezirow, J. (1997). Transformative learning: Theory to practice. *New Directions for Adult and Continuing Education*, 1997(74), 5–12.
11. Arab, M., Ghavami, B., Akbari Lakeh, M., Yaghmaie, M., & Hosseini-Zijoud, S. M. (2015). Learning theory: Narrative review. *International Journal of Medical Reviews*, 2(3), 291–295.
12. Vygotsky, L. (2011). *Interaction between learning and development*. Linköpings Universitet.
13. Torre, D. M., Daley, B. J., Sebastian, J. L., & Elnicki, D. M. (2006). Overview of current learning theories for medical educators. *American Journal of Medicine*, 119(10), 903–907.
14. Kusurkar, R., & ten Cate, O. (2013). AM last page: Education is not filling a bucket, but lighting a fire: Self determination theory and motivation in medical students. *Academic Medicine*, 88(6), 904.
15. Schön, D. A. (1987). *Educating the reflective practitioner: Toward a new design for teaching and learning in the professions*. Jossey-Bass.
16. General Medical Council. (2012). *Leadership and management for all doctors*. GMC. https://www.gmc-uk.org/professional-standards/professional-standards-for-doctors/leadership-and-management-for-all-doctors
17. Mamede, S., van Gog, T., Moura, A. S., de Faria, R. M., Peixoto, J. M., Rikers, R. M., & Schmidt, H. G. (2012). Reflection as a strategy to foster medical students' acquisition of diagnostic competence. *Medical Education*, 46(5), 464–472.
18. Mukhalalati, B. A., & Taylor, A. (2019). Adult learning theories in context: A quick guide for healthcare professional educators. *Journal of Medical Education and Curricular Development*, 6, 2382120519840332.
19. Continuing Professional Development. (2021). *General Medical Council*. Retrieved from https://www.gmc-uk.org/education/standards-guidance-and-curricula/guidance/continuing-professional-development.
20. Manley, K., Martin, A., Jackson, C., & Wright, T. (2018). A realist synthesis of effective continuing professional development (CPD): A case study of healthcare practitioners' CPD. *Nurse Education Today*, 69, 134–141.
21. Stolzenburg, J. U., Schwaibold, H., Bhanot, S. M., Rabenalt, R., Do, M., Truss, M., ... Anderson, C. (2005). Modular surgical training for endoscopic extraperitoneal radical prostatectomy. *BJU International*, 96(7), 1022–1027.

35

Why errors happen

Errors in different specialities vary. In general practice, the errors resulting in litigation often relate to failure to diagnose or refer, while in orthopaedics, they tend to involve surgical complications. In obstetrics, mistiming and misinterpretation (of CTG for example) are the common causes of claims. However, it is very rare that only one category of error will occur in one speciality. The same themes can be found across specialities with only the specific equipment or products varying.

Valuable lessons can be drawn from the errors that are made across the board. Changes to the law can also cause an increase in errors or expose practitioners to allegations that previously would not have been made. For example, since the landmark Montgomery decision, the incidence of consent-related claims has increased. Woodlands hospitals and clinics are increasingly finding themselves vicariously liable for the actions of individual practitioners they engaged solely on a contractor basis.

The nature of errors will also evolve as technological progress is made. For instance, an analysis of 1,000 cases brought in the 1990s against GPs who were members of the MPS found that 19% were due to medication or prescribing errors.[1] Such errors should be on the decline due to the use of computer generation of prescriptions and the inherent safety guards therein protecting against incorrect dosages and iatrogenic adverse drug reactions. Yet, claims regarding remote consultations or reliance on apps that monitor blood sugar levels in diabetics may increase.

The way in which clinicians communicate is also crucial. Failure to communicate clearly, whether with patients or colleagues, can result in claims. Clear communication is key for effecting valid consent, but it is also important for managing patient expectations, as too often, patients have unrealistic views of the outcome of surgery, which in turn leads to claims.

As referred to above, diagnostic errors still play a large part in patient harm, dissatisfaction and litigation. As doctors, we are putting ourselves forward as highly qualified professionals who are trained to make a correct diagnosis. Failing in this can potentially be a breach of duty, but making a wrong diagnosis is not inherently a breach of duty. As long as the thought process was a rational one

DOI: 10.1201/9781003179351-44

that can be justified and supported by a reasonable body of professional opinion, then the diagnostic error itself is acceptable. The traditional model of diagnosis is one of initial collection of information with the history and examination. This is followed by deductive steps to reach the diagnosis or a shortlist of diagnoses.

A diagnostic model formulated by Elstein et al. 25 years ago recognised that the clinician often formulates a putative diagnosis very early on in the consultation.[2] The doctor then recurrently and iteratively tests this and some other possibilities throughout the consultation.[3] The initial hypotheses, usually made up of three or four possible frequent and mundane diagnoses, are usually formulated before much data gathering has occurred. Experienced clinicians will have a gut instinct as to what the pathology might be, and their years of experience will rapidly tunnel the diagnosis to a list of a few potentials. Often, in secondary care, the diagnostic process is targeted as proving or disproving the diagnosis presented in the referral, which can result in bias.

We undergo intensive training at medical school; however, the value of the apprenticeship part of training cannot be overestimated. This vital part of supervised training usually involves the development of strategies and heuristic models that lay the foundations for diagnostic pathways.

The diagnostic process can comprise many parts, as listed below, and each individual clinician will voluntarily or subconsciously prioritise and deprioritise certain cognitive pathways.

- Spot diagnoses
- Self-labelling
- Presenting complaint
- Pattern recognition trigger
- Restricted rule-outs
- Stepwise refinement
- Probabilistic reasoning
- Pattern recognition fit
- Clinical prediction rule
- Known diagnosis
- Further tests ordered
- Test of treatment
- Test of time

Murtagh (1990) described this diagnostic thought process as 'restricted rule-out'.[4]

Both to protect ourselves against litigation and to protect the patient from harm, it makes sense that within a differential diagnosis, the condition at the top of the list should not be the most probable but the condition that we cannot afford to miss.

After forming an initial impression of the illness, the next step is to gather information refining the possibilities by iteratively testing the various diagnoses. We should satisfy ourselves that we can discount the diagnosis that we cannot afford to miss. This must be a conscious and well-documented process.

The diagnosis refinement process involves fitting the presentation to a pattern, which will provide a diagnosis. Care should be taken not to take the diagnosis and then select the presenting features that fit with that diagnosis.

The problem with medicine is that we will err. We are paid and trained to use probabilistic reasoning to ensure that we use NHS resources sparingly; thus, GPs act as gatekeepers to prevent too many patients being referred to secondary care services. Meanwhile, secondary care is burdened by budgets, which restrict investigations and limit resources. Of the thousands of patients a clinician will see in their lifetime, they will likely see a patient with a 1 in 10,000 chance of a certain condition. A rare condition will be seen somewhere by someone, and it will defy probabilistic reasoning. Unfortunately, reliance on probabilistic reasoning is not in itself an adequate defence when faced with a patient with that rare condition that was missed. Clinicians must factor in probabilistic reasoning but also have cognitive safeguards to prevent missing red flags.

Despite the downsides of pure reliance on probabilistic reasoning, it is an invaluable tool to help focus the mind and determine the shortlist of diagnoses. In the last 20 years, there has been more information about the predictive value of symptoms of particular conditions in certain age groups. Much of these data come from secondary care studies (A&E or specialist clinics), as these populations are highly selected groups that have already been through the filter of GP diagnostic acumen.

Increasingly, however, we have primary care data obtained from interrogating anonymised computer data uploaded from primary care clinical systems, such as the General Practice Research Database. These data filter into the computer systems in primary care and should be paid attention to. If they are ignored – which is entirely reasonable, as in the end, they are simply data to guide and assist – there should be a specific reason behind it, and this should be documented.

For example, in primary care, the likelihood that a 65-year-old man with an unexplained haemoglobin of 11.5 g/dL and low ferritin has colorectal cancer is about 6.5%.[5] If the clinician is faced with that scenario but does not choose to refer the patient, then it is necessary to document a definitive reason. In a courtroom, the reality is that the clinician will be challenged and likely found wanting if they cannot provide a rationale for discounting the notion that the patient had colorectal cancer.

The vast amount of data we are now able to collect facilitates the development of clinical prediction rules (CPRs), which are increasingly part of the diagnostic armament and easily accessed via our computer systems. It is important to realise that CPRs are validated and developed in specific population groups and that those validated in secondary care may not always be entirely applicable to primary care. This nuance may not be appreciated in a court of law; thus, caution should be exercised when choosing to ignore them.

A diagnosis is not always essential, and a negative finding (e.g. 'it is not cardiac chest pain') will suffice. Sometimes, we must refine the diagnosis with further tests, such as X-rays, blood tests and urinalysis. It is no longer the case that we should only test if it will change management. Rather, testing comes hand in hand with an action plan. Therefore, we need to consider how we will act upon the results from a blood test. For instance, what is the next step if the C-reactive protein (CRP) is high? Which diagnoses will that refute, and which will it propel up the diagnostic ladder? Failure to act on a blood test result can sometimes be worse than failing to arrange the blood test in the first place.

REFERENCES

1. Silk, N. (2000). What went wrong in 1000 negligence claims. *Health Care Risk Report*, November 2000:13:6.
2. Elstein, A. S., & Schwartz, A. (2000). Clinical problem solving and diagnostic decision making: selective review of the cognitive literature. *BMJ*, 2002 Mar 23;324(7339), 729–32. doi: 10.1136/bmj.324.7339.729.
3. Norman, G. R., & Eva, K. W. (2010). Diagnostic error and clinical reasoning. *Medical Education*, 44, 94–100.
4. Murtagh (1990) - Heneghan C, Glasziou P, Thompson M, Rose P, Balla J, Lasserson D, Scott C, Perera R. Diagnostic strategies used in primary care. *BMJ*. 2009 Apr 20;338:b946.
5. Hamilton, W., Lancashire, R., Sharp. D., Peters, T. J., Cheng, K.K., & Marshall, T. (2008) The importance of anaemia in diagnosing colorectal cancer: a case-control study using electronic primary care records. *Br J Cancer*. Jan 29;98(2), 323–7.

36

Errors and cognitive bias

Human factors for errors are the focus of this chapter. Much research into cognitive reasoning has been conducted to try and determine how and why errors occur. If we can identify common cognitive biases that lead to errors, we can devise strategies and safety nets to mitigate them.

A missed diagnosis, like many errors resulting in harm, is often the result of a sequence of factors that propagate the problem and result in final harm. With misdiagnoses, these are usually not physical errors or errors in data collection but one or more common cognitive errors. All clinicians use cognitive biases, which may lead to the incorrect weighting of evidence.

Cognitive error is pervasive in clinical practice. Up to 75% of errors in medical practice are thought to be cognitive in origin, and errors in cognition have been identified in all steps of the diagnostic process, including information gathering, association triggering, context formulation, processing and verification.[1, 2]

Cognitive biases, also known as heuristics, are cognitive shortcuts that we all use to aid our decision making. A heuristic can be thought of as a cognitive rule of thumb or unwritten guideline that we subconsciously apply to complex situations to make decision making easier and more efficient.

Ironically, a lack of insight into one's own bias is common, demonstrated by doctors who describe themselves as 'excellent' decision-makers and 'free from bias' subsequently scoring poorly in formal test batteries.[3, 4] Therefore, those of us who feel we are immune from bias are likely the ones who need to reflect upon our decision-making processes the most.

An increasingly established framework for understanding the decision-making process is the dual process theory. This theory considers thought processes as type 1 or type 2.[5, 6] This is akin to fast- or slow-twitch muscles. Type 1 thinking is a fast, intuitive, pattern recognition-driven method of problem solving, which places a low cognitive burden on the user and allows the making of fast and accurate decisions, effectively working on autopilot.

By contrast, type 2 thinking is a slower and more methodical and thoughtful process. Type 2 thinking may place a higher cognitive strain on the user but allows them to appraise data more critically and look beyond patterns, and it is potentially more suitable for complex problem solving.

DOI: 10.1201/9781003179351-45

In an ideal world, we would utilise type 2 thinking for all of our important clinical decisions. However, our busy work environments make this an impossible burden. We inevitably combine both thought processes yet train for years to try and develop type 1 thinking to allow ourselves to process and act upon patient data in a fast and efficient manner. However, type 1 thinking is inherently vulnerable to unconscious bias, as it is an unconscious process in itself.

Different types of biases in medical practice include:

- *Anchoring bias*: Placing emphasis on salient features too early in the diagnostic process, with a failure to adjust the initial impression in light of new information. For example, a child presents to a doctor with abdominal pain, and the mother explains at the outset that there are school examinations pending and the child is stressed. This may lead to an early impression of non-organic abdominal pain, which would 'anchor' in place and fail to be swayed by the purely clinical features.

- *Availability bias*: The subconscious disposition to consider diagnoses that more readily come to mind, often dictated by recent experiences. If a disease has not been seen for a long time or is less common, it may be missed. If a clinician has recently attended a seminar on a specific condition or had a previous missed diagnosis, they are more likely to erroneously settle on that diagnosis and give it excessive weighting. For instance, a GP is facing litigation for a missed diagnosis of DVT, and PE will heighten the fear of further missed DVTs and prompt excessive investigations in low-risk patients.

- *Confirmation bias*: The tendency to look for evidence confirming a diagnosis rather than searching for evidence to refute it. Diagnosticians tend to interpret the information gained during a consultation to fit their preconceived diagnosis rather than the converse. With short appointment times, this strategy is inevitable and in the majority of situations is beneficial to ensure focused and efficient diagnosis. However, it is risky in isolation. For example, a patient is non-specifically unwell, and a CRP is taken. This comes back high and is used as a determinant that the patient has an infection rather than prompting a search for other causes of raised CRP.

- *Conjunction bias*: The incorrect belief that the probability of multiple events being true is greater than a single event. This relates to Occam's razor, where a simple and unifying explanation is statistically more likely than multiple disparate explanations. For instance, a patient with joint pains, dry eyes and mouth and raised inflammatory markers is likely to have a systemic inflammatory process rather than osteoarthritis, an infection and unrelated dry eyes and mouth.

- *Overconfidence bias*: A common tendency to believe that we know more than we do and that our diagnostic skills are perfect. Cockiness is an inherent problem that can result in problems. Furthermore, this form of bias can negate all future opportunities to change a diagnosis. This can be augmented by anchoring and availability biases. For example, a consultant makes a definitive diagnosis of normal pressure glaucoma on optic disc appearance, and then, the patient continues to lose vision. Eventually, they are found to have a space-occupying lesion compressing the optic nerve.

- *Representativeness bias*: Restraining decision making along pattern restraint recognition, which may miss atypical diseases. Misinterpreting the likelihood of an event considering both the key similarities to its parent population, and the individual characteristics that define that event. This can be seen in a man who has classic symptoms of a heart attack, is anxious and whose breath smells of alcohol. The latter details have no bearing on the likelihood of a heart attack nor do they alter the degree to which he is a member of his risk demographic, but they can distract and decrease the diagnostic pickup.

- *Search-satisfying bias*: Ceasing to look for further information or alternative diagnoses when the first plausible solution is found. Within the time-pressured environments doctors work in, this is an ever-increasing source of bias. A clinical example is assessing a short-of-breath patient in casualty and diagnosing pneumonia but missing their heart failure, which exacerbates their dyspnoea.

- *Diagnostic momentum bias*: Once diagnostic labels are attached to a patient, they can gather momentum and make it harder to change course. They become fixed in the clinical record, and subsequent clinicians can simply propagate the diagnosis rather than question it when faced with disparate features. The typical example is a diagnosis made by a consultant and then supported and propagated unquestioningly by the junior doctors despite atypical features developing, such as fixating on a previously assigned label of 'possible pulmonary embolism' and organising CT imaging for a patient who may have subsequent results that suggest otherwise (e.g. positive blood cultures the following day).

- *Framing bias*: Pervasive in clinical practice and often seen in the field of radiology. It occurs when a clinician reacts in a specific way dependent upon how the information is presented. For instance, an MRI is requested querying a cerebellar abnormality. The cerebellum is reported as being normal, but a pituitary tumour is missed. The radiologist focuses on the area they are asked about and fails to assess the scan as a whole.

- *Omission bias*: A tendency towards inaction grounded in the principle of do no harm. It is avoidance of active intervention to alter disease progress and the incorrect acceptance of any deterioration as natural history rather than clinician inaction. A tendency towards action rather than inaction. Often, this is the easiest course but can result in patient dissatisfaction if it is the wrong course of action. 'You should have done something to spare me 3 years of pain'.

- *Premature closure bias*: Akin to diagnostic momentum bias. The diagnosis is made, and the game is won. No further thought is given to the condition and the case is closed. All further effort is directed to treatment rather than formulation of the diagnosis.

- *Hindsight bias*: The inability to realistically appraise past events once the outcome becomes known. We continue to develop and grow as clinicians. We should always strive to learn from our errors and those of others. The appraisal process should allow us to develop and prevent future hindsight bias; however, this can result in availability bias and over-investigations.

- *Triage-cueing bias*: Either through patient self-diagnosis or within the pre-referral triage systems of the NHS, the patient is sent in a particular direction and may start the process of diagnostic momentum. Referral to a transient ischaemic attack (TIA) clinic may facilitate discounting of a TIA as the cause of the patient's symptoms but will not determine the underlying cause.

- *Visceral bias*: We all warm to some patients more than others. Aggressive or confrontational patients will get our backs up, but those are the ones who are most likely to complain if an error occurs. This bias relates to the first impression on meeting the patient. It may generate positive or negative feelings, which may affect decision making.

- *Zebra retreat bias*: Refers to the natural reticence to consider a rare diagnosis, even though it is the most likely. 'It cannot be x, as the patient is only 20 years old'. The need to exclude the most serious condition is paramount, and retreating from a diagnosis because it is unlikely will inevitably lead to harm and misdiagnosis for some clinicians (and patients) somewhere at some time. The laws of probability apply to us all.

SOLUTIONS

Cognitive bias is prevalent and a source of significant errors. As health care professionals, we must recognise our fallibility and put in place personal or systemic processes to mitigate the risks.

There is no quick fix. We work in a pressured environment, and though many of these biases are found to be causative of errors, they are also vital processes in our clinical practice. We cannot set aside our training and our gut feeling for fear of bias. Pattern recognition is a vital tool for us. We are supposed to try and make definitive diagnoses in order to move the process forward and develop management strategies.

In addition, we have demanding patients who want action to remedy their problems.

We do not have enough time to bring them back for endless tests that may refute or confirm their preliminary diagnosis. We also need to trust our colleagues, and rather than revisit every diagnosis from scratch, we should be guided by the previous diagnosis. Expecting a clinician to ditch all of these bedrock features of our clinical practice is unreasonable.

The first step in correcting a problem is recognising it. The only way to do this is to set ego aside and realise that we are fallible. Experienced clinicians have been practising medicine successfully by utilising all of the techniques we label as biases for many years. They rarely fail them, and in the vast majority of situations, they are correct. However, they are also likely to be the most set in their ways. They will lock in on a diagnosis and fail to question themselves and reconsider the diagnosis.

We are all aware of the need for reflection, and we routinely reflect on learning opportunities and clinical errors after the fact. It is vital that we reflect on our practice on an ongoing basis and realise that we are prone to errors. Recognising that and having insight is vital to prevent future errors.

As the main tool for preventing cognitive bias and errors, metacognition is a reflective approach to problem solving that involves stepping back from the immediate problem to examine and reflect on the thinking process behind a diagnosis or a management plan. It is the awareness of and insight into one's own thought processes. Such insight forces clinicians to ask themselves 'what else could this be, and am I confident that this is the correct diagnosis?'

Focused teaching in these issues is needed to educate clinicians to recognise where they may be prone to bias. Encouraging a team approach is also vital. If there is diagnostic uncertainty or a fear that a cognitive error has occurred, then asking a colleague's opinion is a low-stress way of getting an objective opinion. Their understanding of the potential for bias will allow an objective assessment of the decision-making process. From a medicolegal perspective, getting a second opinion shows clinical insight and emphasises the reasonableness of our actions.

The best strategy to avoid diagnostic errors is also the most unrealistic and unachievable in modern medical practice. Slowing down is the ideal solution. This allows the diagnostician to transition into type 2 thinking, reflect more critically on the data and ultimately make fewer errors.[6, 7] When faced with deliberate availability bias, medical students who were forced to slowly deliberate performed better, and diagnostic accuracy was shown to improve by simply slowing cognition in two other studies.[8, 9]

With increasing demands, how can the clinician be expected to slow down? Unfortunately, courts do not take into account how busy the clinic was or how far behind schedule we were. Any case is considered in the cold light of day, and 'I only have ten minutes for each patient' or 'my clinic was massively overbooked' is unfortunately given short shrift.

Checklists and protocols are important debiasing strategies that may facilitate and sometimes challenge the diagnostic thought process. Software can assist clinicians in flagging common diagnoses and pointing to protocols. Checklists are used to good effect in any industry to prevent errors.

Ultimately, cognitive bias is a major contributor to medical errors and is underrepresented in education and neglected in clinical practice. Clinicians need to be aware of it and constantly challenge and double-check themselves. Clinicians do not have to do this in isolation, however, and it is vital that systems and teams are in place to recognise and mitigate these biases.

It is unrealistic to expect doctors to abandon the strategies they use regularly and that are often valued as good skills simply because they may be the source of bias. However, doctors should recognise that these tried-and-tested skills they pride themselves on may result in bias and diagnostic errors. We should all lower our threshold for considering the likelihood of cognitive bias in the hope of rec ognising it sooner and remedying it before harm occurs.

Slowing down is impossible, but setting aside details of a patient we are unsure of in order to consider them at the end of our clinic when we have time to engage our type 2 thinking is a sensible precaution. Asking for advice or a second opinion is another tool that should be used more frequently.

Klein et al.[4] summarised rules for decision making, namely:

- Slow down.
- Be aware of base rates for your differentials.
- Consider what data are truly relevant.
- Actively seek alternative diagnoses. Do not be afraid of questioning yourself or others.
- Ask questions to disprove your hypothesis.
- Remember, you are often wrong. Consider the immediate implications of this and remedy this early.

Achieving these goals may be impossible, but the attempt should still be made to avoid problems for ourselves and potentially prevent harm to our patients.

REFERENCES

1. Kassirer, J. P., & Kopelman, R. I. (1989). Cognitive errors in diagnosis: Instantiation, classification, and consequences. *American Journal of Medicine*, 86, 433–41.
2. Graber, M. L., Franklin, N., & Gordon, R. (2005). Diagnostic error in internal medicine. *Archives of Internal Medicine*, 165, 1493–1499.
3. Hershberger, P. J., Part, H. M., Markert, R. J., Cohen, S. M., & Finge, W. W. (1994). Development of a test of cognitive bias in medical decision making. *Academic Medicine*, 69, 839–842.
4. Klein, J. G. (2005). Five pitfalls in decisions about diagnosis and prescribing. *BMJ*, 330, 781–783.
5. Kahneman, D. (2003). Maps of bounded rationality: psychology for behavioural economics. *American Economic Review*, 93, 1449–1475.
6. Kahneman, D. (2011). *Thinking, Fast and Slow* (1st ed.). Farrar, Straus and Giroux.
7. Croskerry, P. (2003). The importance of cognitive errors in diagnosis and strategies to minimize them. *Academic Medicine*, 78, 775–8024.
8. Mamede, S., van Gog, T., van den Berge, K., Rikers, R. M. J. P., van Saase, J. L. C. M., van Guldener, C., & Schmidt, H. G. (2010). Effect of availability bias and reflective reasoning on diagnostic accuracy among internal medicine residents. *JAMA*, 304, 1198–1203.
9. Schmidt, H. G., Mamede, S., van den Berge, K., van Gog, T., van Saase, J. L. C. M., & Rikers, R. M. J. P. (2014). Exposure to media information about a disease can cause doctors to misdiagnose similar-looking clinical cases. *Academic Medicine*, 89, 285–291.

37

Improving diagnosis

The causes of diagnostic errors are multifactorial, but some of the most common are cognitive and knowledge-based, such as decision-making biases, heuristics and misjudgements; lack of knowledge; technical errors; and communication failure. No matter the cause, the result is the same: a delayed or missed diagnosis that costs the patient their time, suffering and sometimes their lives.

For doctors, the resulting complaints and/or potential litigation are also extremely stressful. There is the risk of facing allegations of professional misconduct and clinical negligence as well as guilt if a wrong diagnosis leads to harm or loss of life. Either way, this is a scenario we want to avoid.

Unfortunately, diagnostic errors are among the costliest and most potentially devastating medical errors, and they occur frequently. In settings ranging from primary care to high-level tertiary care, these are prevalent. In the past decade, diagnostic errors have been identified as a serious problem in the medical literature.

According to the NHS Resolution, in 2018/19, there were 10,678 new clinical negligence claims in the NHS.[1] While the numbers were comparatively low considering the high number of patients served by the NHS, the fact remains that many missed and late diagnoses go undetected. According to Elliott et al., there are 237 million errors each year in medication alone, 71% of which occur in primary care.[2] No accurate data exist that can robustly identify the rate of true errors; however, according to some studies, 70% of all medical errors are diagnostic errors.[3]

The consequences of a missed or wrong diagnosis vary based on the speciality, level of hospital (primary/secondary/tertiary), system conditions, etc.

According to a study focusing on emergency medicine, between 2013 and 2015, there were 5,412 cases reported for diagnostic errors.[4] The numbers themselves may not be among the highest within specialities; however, given the nature of the diseases and conditions people visit EDs with, the consequences are graver than dermatological diagnostic errors, for example.

Most missed diagnoses in EDs are myocardial infarction, intracranial bleeds and fractures, of which hip and spine fractures are the most common types. Suffice to say, missing these diagnoses can lead to patient death and permanent

DOI: 10.1201/9781003179351-46

damage. Naturally, the clinical negligence claims and potential payouts can be significant. The hospital in which a patient is attended to is a factor as well. Although diagnostic errors have been discussed primarily in hospital settings, research suggests that they also occur frequently in primary care environments.

The most common types of diagnostic errors are misdiagnosis (e.g. appendicitis), missed diagnosis (e.g. melanoma) and delayed diagnosis (e.g. lung cancer). An individual's cognitive abilities play a role in diagnostic errors, in addition to system factors affecting patient safety, which can sometimes contribute to these errors more than individual factors do.

A very common cause is flaws in clinical reasoning. It is difficult to identify a correct diagnosis when a patient's symptoms and signs do not conform to expectations. Our ability to catalogue all possible disease presentations has not kept pace with our expanding knowledge of diseases. Additionally, unanticipated presentations may be due to diseases we have yet to discover or understand or to nuances within conditions we see frequently.

According to Wellbery, flaws in reasoning are often caused by the internal cognitive biases of professionals.[5] Cognitive biases are mostly heuristics or shortcuts physicians use to reach a diagnosis. Most are tried-and-true methods developed through a physician's experience. The risk of this method is that some diagnoses will fall through the patterns, which may have been easy to spot without the bias. In fact, according to some authors, '75% of errors in internal medicine are thought to be cognitive in origin'.[6]

Cognitive errors are discussed in depth in Chapter 36. Cognitive biases, by their nature, are hard to detect.

A CASE IN POINT[7]

A female patient in her 50s reported to the hospital with a rapidly progressing weakness while visiting Mexico. She first developed mild muscle pain, which progressed to leg weakness and then the inability to stand. After hospitalisation, the weakness moved upwards towards her upper extremities and neck. She was left unable to move her hands and legs but had a stable respiratory status. There was bilateral severe proximal worse than distal weakness in all limbs. She was found to have long-term facial paraesthesia and dry mouth.

While an inpatient in Mexico, a visiting professor was asked to diagnose the patient. After taking her history, he diagnosed her condition as acute trichinosis. The rationale behind his diagnosis was that the patient was visiting Mexico and she could have contracted trichinosis, which was consistent with the typical proximal worse than distal weakness of the limbs, sparing the respiratory muscle and face and preserving the reflexes. At first glance, the diagnosis seemed accurate.

However, a framing bias was in effect. The diagnosis was based on the first information that was provided, which was that the patient was in Mexico when her conditions first developed. The professor was also provided her blood test results, which showed she had abnormal serum potassium, high ESR, rheumatoid factors and Sjögren syndrome A and B antibodies. The lab results pointed to the correct diagnosis, which was hypokalaemia due to distal renal tubular acidosis caused by Sjögren's.

Another case study showed a common scenario at the NHS: anchoring and premature closure. As physicians are pressed for time, they will often diagnose based on the chief complaints given by the patient. For example, when a patient, obese with normal to high blood sugar, presented with a rash below their arms, it was reasonably diagnosed as intertrigo. The diagnosis was highly likely, so the GP would probably have asked them to return if the rash did not disappear.

However, the patient had pain in their joints, which was not mentioned in their first visit. The patient later went to another doctor, who diagnosed them with arthritis and referred them to a rheumatologist. It was at the rheumatologist where the correct diagnosis was discovered: erythema migrans associated with Lyme disease.[8] The first two doctors focused on only one symptom, and the systemic condition eluded them.

Nevertheless, cognitive biases, or heuristics to be exact, are an effective tool to improve diagnosis, even though they may lead to errors. There are hundreds of possible clinical diagnoses for each symptom. To reach the most probable one, a clinician needs to be able to read the patterns of a patient's symptoms through training/repetition, which is aided by heuristics.

Heuristics save time and resources and are undeniably necessary to be a good health care professional.

Making decisions based on intuition or previous knowledge is how we make diagnoses and clinical judgements on a day-to-day basis, unless there are any indications to not do so, such as sensitive cases or worsening patient conditions. According to Rottman, most physicians use Bayesian reasoning to reach a diagnosis.[9]

Bayesian reasoning is simple: 'the most important determinants of the posterior probability of disease are the prior probability and the test properties'.[10] This means that the known probability of a disease and the test results/symptoms shown by a patient determine the probability of that patient having the disease. For example, if a patient has pox-like spots, they may be either chickenpox or smallpox. But the doctor already knows the chances of chickenpox are higher than smallpox; hence, coupled with the symptoms, the most probable disease the patient has is chickenpox. Although the use of Bayesian reasoning is not deliberate, it is intuitive and an inherent part of heuristics.

The conclusions doctors reach based on their own knowledge and experience are usually more likely to be correct than those based on data, such as prevalence rates. Therefore, knowledge-based decisions cannot be cast away, but they will be wrong sometimes.

As mentioned in an earlier chapter, cognitive psychologists propose two types of thinking that portray the duality in the diagnostic process. One type of thinking process is intuitive, fast and based on patterns or 'rapid autonomous processes', called type 1 thinking. The other type is based on 'distinctive higher order reasoning processes' or on the analysis of available data and logical reasoning. This type is called type 2 thinking.[10, 11]

Type 1 thinking refers to fast, automatic, intuitive and effortless thinking. These types of decisions are based on mental shortcuts or heuristics. The diagnosis is made using the physician's experience and pattern recognition (i.e. they have seen this before). Type 2 thinking refers to slower, more analytical and more effortful thinking. The diagnosis is based on methodical exploration and patient examination. It often involves ordering further tests, reviewing current medications and consulting with colleagues or a specialist. To reach a correct diagnosis, we need both.

Metacognition is a practical approach to using both systems. The theory of metacognition can be defined as 'the capacity for self-reflection on the process of thinking and self-regulation in monitoring decision making'.[12] In other words, it is the use of type 2 thinking to reassess or reflect on the decisions reached with type 1 thinking.

This type of self-reflection can be used by clinicians to help them make more accurate decisions about diagnoses and treatments. The concept of metacognition is not new. Many proponents and researchers advocate it as a critical skill for medical professionals to develop. The idea behind this approach to clinical reasoning is that clinicians must develop the ability to reflect on their own thinking processes. The practitioner must be able to thoroughly examine the steps taken prior to, during and after an event to accurately diagnose a patient's problem.

According to Heneghan et al., the diagnostic process can be divided into three steps: *initiation of diagnostic hypotheses, refinement of the diagnostic hypotheses and defining the final diagnosis.*[13] Dividing it gives more control over each step and a specific set of tools to employ at each step.

The first stage is the initiation of the diagnosis. It occurs within the first few minutes of consultation. Some strategies that can be used in this stage are:

- **Spot diagnosis**: That is the unconscious recognition of non-verbal patterns or symptoms; for example, a teenage patient coming to the dermatologist with several large areas of acne or a patient visiting their GP with a barking cough. Physicians of the associated speciality can identify the patterns shown by the symptoms immediately. Sixty-three per cent of these conditions do not need further diagnostic tests, as doctors would recognise them as easily as they would their relatives, according to Sackett et al.'s 'Auntie Minnie' phenomenon.[14]

- **Self-labelling**: A patient may tell the physician what they think they have. Self-labelling may be accurate in some cases but can result in framing bias errors. If a patient has chronic conditions, for example, or recurring infections, taking their opinion into account increases the probability of a correct diagnosis. They also use 'Dr Google' to aid in their self-diagnoses.

- **Chief complaint**: The initial diagnosis or differential diagnosis should always address the chief complaint of the patient. However, the associated complaints may also point to the correct diagnosis, and it is the clinician's professional obligation to tease out those associated symptoms through questioning. For example, to a patient, 'feeling thirsty more often' or 'having to use the bathroom more' is not as significant as the recurring infections/ulcers they have, but these lead to a potential diagnosis of diabetes.

The second stage is the refinement stage. In this stage, the clinician refines the choices or ideas they made. The strategies for this step are:

- **Restricted rule-outs**: Murtagh's restricted rule-out is an excellent tool to rule out disorders/diseases until we are left with the most probable one. In the diagnostic process, a restricted rule-out is a strategy that lists the possible diagnoses, which are eliminated in stepwise fashion afterwards. The eliminations are based on test results, further symptoms, disease progression/evolution, etc. For example, the patient's clinical features might fit an initial diagnosis, but the laboratory result is inconsistent with it, resulting in the removal of the diagnosis.

- **Stepwise refinement**: A stepwise refinement is a process in which the initial complaint is narrowed down to an anatomical site or pathological process. Next, the possibilities are eliminated stepwise until the correct diagnosis is reached. For example, a red and itchy eye may be local or systemic. Once the root cause is confirmed as local, such as conjunctivitis, the next step is to determine whether the conjunctivitis is infectious or allergic.

- **Pattern recognition**: Recognising the patterns of symptoms and the patterns of previous patients is not only helpful for diagnosis but also prepares a physician for the possible outcomes of diseases and treatments.

- **Clinical prediction rules**: These are handy for new doctors and are often available as part of the EPR software. They are essentially patterns associated with diseases formalised with repetitive use. Clinical rules and patterns established by experienced clinicians are usually well tested and reliable. Streptococcal sore throat rules, depression HAD scores, DVT (Wells rule) and the ABCDE of emergency patient management are excellent examples of existing rules that apply well and can help reach reasonable goals.[15, 16]

The final stage of diagnosis is to fine-tune the narrowed-down list and choose one diagnosis that is the most likely. Often, this is done in the clinician's head; however, should the diagnosis be wrong, it is important that the thought process is documented clearly. If there is no evidence that other diagnoses were scrutinised and excluded, then we leave ourselves open to allegations of 'failed to consider'.

As stated earlier, a clinician owes a duty of care to the patient to consider all potential diagnoses, but sometimes, they will pick the incorrect one. By itself, making a wrong diagnosis is not a breach of duty as long as it was reasonable to do so, and the same decision would have been reached by a reasonable body of medical opinion.

The strategies that help physicians achieve this last refinement step with minimal mistakes are:

- **Tests**: If the diagnosis is still unclear after the previous strategies have been exhausted, then the best course of action is to order more tests. While these tests are being arranged, it is reasonable to commence treatment for the most harmful condition on the differential diagnosis list. More information narrows down or directs the possibilities, and the potential correct diagnosis should be clearer.

- **Known diagnosis**: Treatment can be started after a sufficient idea regarding the disease has been formed, depending on the nature of the disease and the level of certainty required from the physician. If the treating physician is a GP, their job is to suspect an acute condition, start the initial treatment and refer to the closest available secondary care provider. The nature of the disease determines whether an accurate diagnosis is needed or not.

  For example, conjunctivitis caused by different pathogens has the same management, so determining the pathogen type is not needed, unless the symptoms differ from the norm and there is a concern that there is a sight-compromising pathology.[17]

- **Test of treatment and time**: This is a common and efficient strategy used by most physicians to minimise the need to bring patients back on multiple occasions. If we cannot confirm a diagnosis with 100% surety, a strategic move is to commence treatment and place a safety net by asking the patient to return if the symptoms do not subside within a given amount of time.

The treatment may confirm the diagnosis or refute it. It is part of the diagnostic process. For example, giving an inhaler for night cough can be used to confirm or refute a diagnosis of bronchospasm. Diseases that are usually transient can be waited out, given there are no serious symptoms.

For example, a nursery child having acute sensitivity in their palms and feet with soreness of the throat can be assumed to have hand-foot-mouth disease. Most GPs would not advise any treatment apart from sore throat management and waiting for a few days to see whether the condition improves or worsens. As long as there is adequate safety netting that is clearly relayed to the patient, ideally in written form, then even if the diagnosis is wrong, the potential harm is mitigated.

COMPUTER ASSISTANCE

Making a diagnosis is still very much a clinician's job, but computers can make the process easier, safer and more efficient. The use of EPRs in the NHS, for example, allows a doctor to assess all available data of a patient in one place, giving them enough information to reach a differential diagnosis.

The EPR has two major uses. The first is that it was designed to replace the paper-based records that had been kept in hospitals for many years. It involves creating an electronic record for each patient, including their past medical history and the details of their stay in hospital.

The second use of the EPR is that it replaces the paper notes that doctors and other health care professionals use to record their observations about a patient's condition. It improves communication between health professionals and patients and also between different staff members (e.g. hospital doctors and GPs). EPRs are also intended to improve the quality and safety of patient care by providing more up-to-date and accurate information about a patient's condition. Rather than relying on the patient to recall allergies and previous treatments, we can access all their data ourselves.

As health care professionals and patients grow increasingly comfortable with the benefits of technology, remote monitoring, online tools for diagnosis and other options are becoming more popular. Some are available now, while others need more time and research before they can be used daily with complete confidence.

Online directories and apps are accessible and beneficial tools for looking up diagnoses, treatments and doses. Several private practices use software that can automate medication options and doses once given the diagnosis. Some help clinicians think through clinical problems more systematically by offering checklists and questions to ask. Medical websites intended for trainees offer searchable symptoms and their associated conditions for better diagnosis.

Furthermore, several mobile applications have built-in data stores to search symptoms, patterns, examination techniques, drug dose calculators and X-ray analysis tools. There is also a growing interest in artificial intelligence (AI) for medical use these days, and for good reason. AI-powered tools can not only analyse massive amounts of data to generate effective treatment plans but also help to diagnose illnesses and predict disease progression. However, AI-assisted tools are yet to be mass-produced.

The status of these tools is unclear when it comes to medicolegal issues. The ultimate responsibility remains with the health care professional, so it is important to ensure that we are satisfied with the information we access and its use.

REFERENCES

1. Ient, A. (2022, January 4). Clinical negligence numbers steady, but rising costs remain a concern. *NHS Resolution*. Retrieved from https://resolution.nhs.uk/2019/07/11/clinical-negligence-numbers-steady-but-rising-costs-remain-a-concern/.
2. Elliott, R., Camacho, E., Campbell, F., Jankovic, D., St James, M. M., Kaltenthaler, E., ... Faria, R. (2018). Prevalence and economic burden of medication errors in the NHS in England. Rapid evidence synthesis and economic analysis of the prevalence and burden of medication error in the UK. *BMJ Qual Saf*, 30(2), 96–105.

3. Tehrani, A. S. S., Lee, H., Mathews, S. C., Shore, A., Makary, M. A., Pronovost, P. J., & Newman-Toker, D. E. (2013). 25-Year summary of US malpractice claims for diagnostic errors 1986–2010: An analysis from the national practitioner data bank. *BMJ Quality & Safety*, 22(8), 672–680.

4. Hussain, F., Cooper, A., Carson-Stevens, A., Donaldson, L., Hibbert, P., Hughes, T., & Edwards, A. (2019). Diagnostic error in the emergency department: Learning from national patient safety incident report analysis. *BMC Emergency Medicine*, 19(1), 1–9.

5. Wellbery, C. E. (2011). Flaws in clinical reasoning: A common cause of diagnostic error. *American Family Physician*, 84(9), 1042–1048.

6. O'Sullivan, E. D., & Schofield, S. J. (2018). Cognitive bias in clinical medicine. *Journal of the Royal College of Physicians of Edinburgh*, 48(3), 225–231.

7. Vickrey, B. G., Samuels, M. A., & Ropper, A. H. (2010). How neurologists think: A cognitive psychology perspective on missed diagnoses. *Annals of Neurology*, 67(4), 425–433.

8. Wellbery, C. E. (2011). Flaws in clinical reasoning: A common cause of diagnostic error. *American Family Physician*, 84(9), 1042–1048.

9. Rottman, B. M. (2017). Physician Bayesian updating from personal beliefs about the base rate and likelihood ratio. *Memory & Cognition*, 45(2), 270–280.

10. Bours, M. J. (2021). Bayes' rule in diagnosis. *Journal of Clinical Epidemiology*, 131, 158–160.

11. Evans, J. S. B., & Stanovich, K. E. (2013). Dual-process theories of higher cognition: Advancing the debate. *Perspectives on Psychological Science*, 8(3), 223–241.

12. Daniel, K. (2017). *Thinking, fast and slow*. Penguin.

13. Heneghan, C., Glasziou, P., Thompson, M., Rose, P., Balla, J., Lasserson, D., ... Perera, R. (2009). Diagnostic strategies used in primary care. *BMJ*, 338, b946.

14. Sackett, D. L., Haynes, R. B., & Tugwell, P. (1995). *Clinical epidemiology* (1st ed.). Little Brown.

15. Ebell, M. H., Smith, M. A., Barry, H. C., Ives, K., & Carey, M. (2000). Does this patient have strep throat? *JAMA*, 284(22), 2912–2918.

16. Bjelland, I., Dahl, A. A., Haug, T. T., & Neckelmann, D. (2002). The validity of the hospital anxiety and depression scale: An updated literature review. *Journal of Psychosomatic Research*, 52(2), 69–77.

17. Rose, P. W., Harnden, A., Brueggemann, A. B., Perera, R., Sheikh, A., Crook, D., & Mant, D. (2005). Chloramphenicol treatment for acute infective conjunctivitis in children in primary care: A randomised double-blind placebo-controlled trial. *The Lancet*, 366(9479), 37–43.

38

Protecting yourself from litigation

There is no way to fully protect yourself from litigation. It should be taken as part and parcel of being a health care professional. There are however ways we can seek to avoid clinical errors, which are the root cause of litigation, complaints, which are often the precursor for litigation, and, if litigation ensues, we can protect ourselves from adverse findings.

KNOW YOUR STUFF

It is vital that your knowledge base is up to date. You will be judged on the standards in force at the time. You will not be expected to be up to date with the latest scientific developments; however, you will be expected to be up to date with any nationally published guidance and adhere to standard practice. What that standard practice is will be determined by the legal tests that have been discussed earlier in this text. You are not expected to be a 'super doctor' or an 'exceptional nurse' but instead achieve the standard of a reasonable health care professional in the same role.

If there is National Institute for Health and Clinical Excellence (NICE) Guidance in force at the time, then it will be used as a standard to which you should have adhered. It should be noted that adherence to NICE Guidance is not compulsory and indeed the guidance is accompanied by the statement:

This guidance represents the views of NICE and was arrived at after careful consideration of the evidence available. Healthcare professionals are expected to take it fully into account when exercising their clinical judgment. However, the guidance does not override the individual responsibility of healthcare professionals to make decisions appropriate to the circumstances of the individual patient in consultation with the patient and/or guardian or carer.

DOI: 10.1201/9781003179351-47

So, there is some wriggle room, and it is not binding; however, if you diverge from such guidance you need to document the reasoning well. Remember that if it does go to court the judge will make the ultimate decision and when he/she is faced with guidance which specifically makes recommendations, and you did not follow it, they may find against you even if others would do the same thing. Remember that the Bolitho Test helped to clarify what was meant by 'a responsible body' of medical opinion by highlighting that the action had to have a 'logical basis'. Therefore a judge may not find that not adhering to scientifically sound guidance is 'logical'.

In most circumstances unless there is a precise reason for not following it no responsible body of medical opinion will support practice that contradicts the NICE Guidance. The reasonable argument of a patient who has come to harm will be that the guidance should have been followed and, if failure to do so resulted in harm, then there will be a valid case for breach of duty.

KNOW LOCAL GUIDELINES

Adherence to local guidelines is vital, and it is the health care professional's obligation to be aware of them. If there is a guidance note which is produced by your own organisation and you do not follow it then there is a clear issue. No responsible body of opinion will support actions which do not adhere to local guidance, and such actions will be very hard to defend. If you are in a managerial role or have a team, then it is important that all members of the team know these local guidelines and adhere to them unless there is a specific reason not to and this is documented.

KEEP UP TO DATE

Engaging in continual professional development (CPD) is central to the work of all health care professionals to deliver high-quality, safe and effective care. CPD can take lots of different forms including formal learning activities and informal learning relevant to your specific role, all with the purpose of continually updating and renewing your knowledge and skills and optimising your evidence-based practice. Health care evolves, and it is important that you are keeping up. This does not mean that you need to be at the forefront of the advance, but you should endeavour to be within the wave behind it by ensuring your practice is consistent with that of your peers.

In the UK CPD is mandated by various professional bodies including the General Medical Council and the Nursing and Midwifery Council.

BE AWARE OF THE COGNITIVE ERRORS THAT ARISE

Chapters 35 and 36 describe various ways in which clinical errors can occur and the underlying cognitive issues that can predispose to them. It is important to recognise that you can err and that you are susceptible to cognitive errors. Be on the lookout for them and try to develop strategies to detect them. Reassess diagnoses regularly and try to think outside the box. If the clinical course is suboptimal, take a step back to assess the reason and to second guess the diagnosis.

HAVE INSIGHT

Insight is vital as a health care professional. Failure to acknowledge and learn from errors is often more concerning than the error itself as it can highlight a concern around future conduct. Stubbornness and refusal to acknowledge an issue/error will quickly polarise the positions and will be more likely to escalate to litigation. Regulatory bodies, management and ultimately the judge will look unfavourably on the health care professional who does not recognise their error and is not willing to learn from it to prevent harm in the future.

RAPPORT WITH PATIENTS

Establishing a rapport with your patient is vital, and this starts from the very first engagement. It can have a positive impact on patient outcomes and patient satisfaction and reduce the risk of medical errors and complaints. Offering an explanation when things have not gone to plan will help reassure the patient that there is no 'cover up' and that their condition has been managed appropriately. Good communication is vital and particularly so when things do not go to plan and there is an error/adverse event.

ROLE OF THE SECOND OPINION

Consider a second opinion early when the management of the patient is not going to plan. This is effectively a mini-Bolam test in that if your colleague agrees with your management then it could be argued that a responsible body of medical opinion supports your practice even though it may simply be another health care professional in the same role as yourself. Explaining to a patient that you have sought a second opinion because their condition is atypical or complex reassures the patient that you are doing the best for them under difficult circumstances and may offer a different perspective on the management plan. It also shows insight as recognising that health care is a team enterprise is vital and none of us are infallible.

ROBUST CONSENT IN SPECIAL CIRCUMSTANCES

Good consent practice is vital, particularly for surgical procedures. It is vital that, if a patient has a specific risk individual to them, it is discussed and documented as otherwise there will be an argument that the consent was not tailored to the individual which it should be. Avoid simply referring to information sheets on the consent form. Try and interact with the consent form to show that you engaged with the consent process and did not simply ask a patient to 'sign the form'.

IF THINGS ARE NOT GOING RIGHT DOCUMENT WELL

Documentation is always an issue; historically this has been related to poor hand-writing but now can be related to failure to adequately complete the electronic patient record. Not ticking a box can be misinterpreted as not having undertaken that part of the examination.

If the patient is not progressing as planned then it is vital that documentation is robust and clear. If there are complications, issues or the potential for a complaint then it is vital that the clinician takes a bit longer with the documentation and makes sure that the clinical record is detailed. Document the differential diagnoses, the treatment options, the discussion with the patient surrounding those treatment options and the rationale behind the eventual management decision.

Always be aware that there may be another health care professional scrutinising those records and determining whether you did consider other diagnoses or options and whether the standard of care you provided was to an acceptable standard. When making decisions document your thinking process and rationale behind those decisions. This will allow other health care professionals to rationalise your practice and can potentially avoid adverse findings. The practice may not be what the 'expert' would have done, but if there is a valid thought process behind the action, even if it was ultimately incorrect, then is it unlikely to be deemed a breach of duty. If the decision has no explanation, then it could be misinterpreted as rash and something that would not be supported by a responsible body of medical opinion.

Avoid the use of new techniques with insufficient training, evidence base or audit.

Ensure appropriate supervision and engagement with junior staff and the wider health care team.

Engage actively with the complaint or investigation process and avoid escalation.

Ultimately, despite every effort, errors, complaints and litigation occur; however, there are strategies that can be adopted to mitigate the risks of harm and the likelihood of escalation or adverse findings.

Index

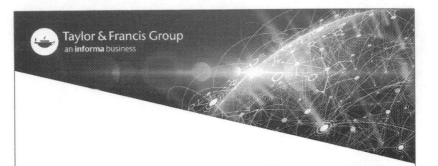

Printed in the United States
by Baker & Taylor Publisher Services